Overcoming Common Problems Series

Selected titles

A full list of titles is available from Sheldon Press,
36 Causton Street, London SW1P 4ST and on our website at
www.sheldonpress.co.uk

101 Questions to Ask Your Doctor
Dr Tom Smith

Asperger Syndrome in Adults
Dr Ruth Searle

Birth Over 35
Sheila Kitzinger

Bulimia, Binge-eating and their Treatment
Professor J. Hubert Lacey, Dr Bryony Bamford
and Amy Brown

Coeliac Disease: What you need to know
Alex Gazzola

Coping Successfully with Prostate Cancer
Dr Tom Smith

Coping with Asthma in Adults
Mark Greener

Coping with Bronchitis and Emphysema
Dr Tom Smith

Coping with Drug Problems in the Family
Lucy Jolin

Coping with Dyspraxia
Jill Eckersley

Coping with Early-onset Dementia
Jill Eckersley

Coping with Envy
Dr Windy Dryden

Coping with Gout
Christine Craggs-Hinton

**Coping with Life's Challenges: Moving on
from adversity**
Dr Windy Dryden

**Coping with Manipulation: When others
blame you for their feelings**
Dr Windy Dryden

Coping with the Psychological Effects of Cancer
Professor Robert Bor, Dr Carina Eriksen
and Ceilidh Stapelkamp

Coping with Rheumatism and Arthritis
Dr Keith Souter

Coping with Snoring and Sleep Apnoea
Jill Eckersley

Coping with Stomach Ulcers
Dr Tom Smith

**Divorce and Separation: A legal guide
for all couples**
Dr Mary Welstead

Dying for a Drink
Dr Tim Cantopher

**Epilepsy: Complementary and alternative
treatments**
Dr Sallie Baxendale

**High-risk Body Size: Take control
of your weight**
Dr Funké Baffour

How to Beat Worry and Stress
Dr David Delvin

How to Develop Inner Strength
Dr Windy Dryden

**How to Lower Your Blood Pressure:
And keep it down**
Christine Craggs-Hinton

**Let's Stay Together: A guide to lasting
relationships**
Jane Butterworth

Living with Fibromyalgia
Christine Craggs-Hinton

**Living with a Problem Drinker:
Your survival guide**
Rolande Anderson

Living with a Stoma
Professor Craig A. White

Living with Tinnitus and Hyperacusis
Dr Laurence McKenna, Dr David Baguley
and Dr Don McFerran

Losing a Parent
Fiona Marshall

Motor Neurone Disease: A family affair
Dr David Oliver

Natural Treatments for Arthritis
Christine Craggs-Hinton

**Overcoming Gambling: A guide for problem
and compulsive gamblers**
Philip Mawer

**The Pain Management Handbook:
Your personal guide**
Neville Shone

Reducing Your Risk of Dementia
Dr Tom Smith

**Therapy for Beginners: How to get the best
out of counselling**
Professor Robert Bor, Sheila Gill and Anne
Stokes

Understanding Traumatic Stress
Dr Nigel Hunt and Dr Sue McHale

When Someone You Love Has Dementia
Susan Elliot-Wright

Overcoming Common Problems

The Pain Management Handbook

Your personal guide

NEVILLE SHONE

sheldon **PRESS**

First published in Great Britain in 2011

Sheldon Press
36 Causton Street
London SW1P 4ST
www.sheldonpress.co.uk

British Library Cataloguing-in-Publication Data
A catalogue record for this book is available from the British Library

ISBN 978-1-84709-142-0
eBook ISBN 978-1-84709-210-6

Typeset by Fakenham Prepress Solutions, Fakenham, Norfolk NR21 8NN
First printed in Great Britain by Ashford Colour Press
Subsequently digitally printed in Great Britain

Produced on paper from sustainable forests

Contents

Acknowledgements

I would like to thank professional colleagues in the UK and the USA for their continuing help and support.

I would also like to thank Joanna Moriarty and Fiona Marshall for encouraging me to put pen to paper again and for their help in seeing this book to fruition. Thanks are also owed to the staff of Sheldon Press for their guidance on technical matters.

I owe a debt of gratitude to all the people with pain I have worked with over the years in Liverpool, Scotland and Spain, who allowed me try out my ideas on them and who trusted me to help them to help themselves. They all survived.

Finally, my thanks to my wife Eve for the sometimes taxing typing – and retyping – job and for acting as my sounding board.

A word from the author

Have you experienced pain for longer than three months? Have you had surgery that has left you with residual pain? Are you undergoing treatment that you feel is not accomplishing anything? Have you been searching for a cure or run the gamut of doctors or hospitals in a fruitless quest for pain relief? Do you feel the doctors have given up on you? Do you feel that the drugs you are taking are damaging your health? Do you feel helpless and that no one believes you have pain? Do you sometimes feel like giving up? Do you feel your pain is changing your personality and no longer recognize yourself?

If so, then it is time for you to take a new approach and learn those skills that are necessary to manage your pain. I did, and so have thousands of others. This book contains everything you need to know . . . to help you smile again.

Note to the reader

None of the ideas, advice and exercises in this book is intended as a substitute for the medical advice of your doctor. Before adopting any of the suggestions in this book, consult your medical practitioner about any condition that may require diagnosis or treatment. Any statements made by the author concerning products and services represent the opinion of the author alone and do not constitute a recommendation or endorsement of any product or service. The author cannot accept any liability arising directly from the use of this book.

Prologue

Even though almost 30 years have passed, the consultant's words still resound in my mind:

You might as well get used to leading a completely restricted life.

The words were chilling. I do not think I heard anything else he said, until his parting words: 'I'll see you again in six months.' My mind was racing as I wondered why he should want to see me again, if he was dismissing me so finally. I was confused. My present activities were almost completely restricted. I struggled to get from one hour to the next without pain, cramps or muscle spasms. I felt extreme pain each time I put my foot to the ground. If I tried to get into my car I was physically sick with the pain. I could barely get through the first course of a meal without getting up from the table to ease the discomfort. My sleep was fitful and disturbed by cramps in my legs, ribs and the long muscles on either side of my spine, and my mind was filled by a succession of negative thoughts. I was in a permanent state of exhaustion. If I went into the garden to try to tidy up, I could dead-head only half a dozen roses before I was forced to retire indoors, defeated by pain.

My appearance in the mirror frightened me. My cheeks were sunken and my face was grey. I was bent over forwards and to one side. I just could not stand up straight. It took me two hours to get showered and dressed in the morning, and when it was done I was exhausted. I was not able to take medication because I was allergic to everything but paracetamol, which did little or nothing to relieve my pain. How had I got into this situation?

Six months earlier I had undergone surgery for the removal of a benign tumour on my spine. On reflection, I think pain had always been with me. I can remember, as a child, lying in bed and experiencing what I can only describe as 'toothache' in my knees and hips. This was dismissed as 'growing pains' that every child had to cope with. I can remember how painful it was to sit upright studying at a desk or table, and I was often told off for wriggling about on dining chairs at mealtimes. I was experiencing intense discomfort. It was not a time to complain about 'trivial' aches and pains and I knew if I did I would not get much sympathy. There was a war on. This was not an unusual attitude to take. Families were preoccupied about how to feed the family at home and worried about the welfare of those away fighting. There was the constant fear of being bombed – or worse.

My mother had been a widow since I was five years old and, to help out with family finances, I went to work. From the age of 9 to 13 I worked on a farm for two hours a day after school and from 8.00 a.m. to 6.00 p.m. on Saturdays, summer and winter, rain or shine. I planted and hoed cabbages, picked Brussels sprouts, peas and potatoes and did whatever else that needed doing, according to the season – and the farmer.

Child labour was not unusual in the 1940s and, as a matter of pride, I did my best to keep up with the adult workers. Incidentally, for my pains, I was paid the princely sum of 10 shillings a week, equivalent to 50p today. After four years I needed to earn more money for books and running shoes, so I became a delivery boy for an ironmonger, where I stayed until I was 17 and preparing for A-levels. With hindsight, this physical work at so young an age did no favours to my immature body. As I got older, I also became involved in athletics and school musicals, in addition to all the other normal activities of a teenager.

My 'growing pains' did not go away and I accepted them as normal. I thought everybody had them. When they bothered me, I thought it was my body telling me to ease off. Studying for exams at school, and later at university, became quite an ordeal. However, I had always been active and achieved well academically. They did not stop me pursuing my career and enjoying a full social life.

Before I reached 30 I began to get back pain, serious enough for me occasionally to take time off work. The back pain was never investigated. The accepted treatment was bed rest for two or three weeks. By this time I was married and had a family of three children; I was fully involved with my work as a university teacher, with family activities and in my hobby of amateur theatre. Candle, both ends? Within the space of a few years the severity of the pain had increased and I found it a struggle to cope with driving to work 25 miles away. By this time I was head of department, leading a team of academics, directing a research project, acting as an external examiner at several universities and undertaking additional teaching work for central and local government organizations.

When I was 44 all this activity and my career came to a sudden end when I suffered a collapse. Life as I knew it was over.

Introduction – The problem reviewed

Many illnesses cause pain or fatigue for a few days or weeks; but chronic pain, as the name suggests, is long lasting. People with chronic pain, that is people who have had their pain for more than three months, share the experience of having a problem that appears to be intractable, in spite of the best efforts of the medical profession. As a result they share feelings of abandonment, anger and even rage, loss, frustration, depression and helplessness – conditions that are serious enough in themselves to merit treatment. These feelings add considerably to the burden of pain. It is the intention of this handbook to make available to people with chronic pain some of the information, knowhow and skills that can enable them to free themselves from their 'prison of pain' and set them on the path towards reconstructing their lives. Even if the pain has gone on for years it is not too late to begin this process.

The chronic pain syndrome causes extreme fatigue, joint and muscle pain and other symptoms. It can strike anywhere but is especially common in the back, head and extremities. The most common conditions that give rise to chronic pain include:

- rheumatoid arthritis and osteoarthritis
- osteoporosis
- spondylitis and spondylosis
- spinal stenosis
- fibromyalgia
- myalgic encephalopathy (ME), also known as chronic fatigue syndrome
- sciatica
- facet joint pain
- ruptured or bulging discs, causing severe back, head or neck pain that can radiate down the arms and legs
- tumours, malignant or non-malignant, which can cause nerve irritation
- multiple sclerosis (MS)

- neuralgia, for example trigeminal neuralgia causing severe facial pain, or postherpetic neuralgia (pain after shingles)
- postoperative adhesions and adhesions following injury
- scar tissue and tissue damage, which can produce nerve irritation leading to prolonged, persistent pain
- cancer pain and pain following cancer treatment.

Pain can continue as residual pain even after an acute problem has been resolved. Phantom limb pain can exist long after an amputation. Sometimes, chronic pain has no physical cause and is thought to be due to emotional and psychological factors such as stress or depression. People who have been told that no reasons can be suggested for their pain, in spite of extensive tests and investigations, are often devastated, feeling that it is being implied that the pain is all in their imagination or that they are malingering.

It is part of British culture to joke about bad backs and to deride those who stay off work with back pain. However, anyone who works in the field of pain management knows and accepts that the pain is real. It is just that the cause is not easily identifiable and results from a complex mix of physical, psychological, emotional and social factors. It may not result from an illness or pathological condition but can be the result of putting muscles under too much tension. For example, from standing or sitting badly for long periods, or from constant repetition of movement, such as in repetitive strain injury. Candidates for this type of problem are people who sit at a desk or checkout for long hours or repeat the same hand movements over and over again every working day. Hairdressing is an occupation that can lead to such problems, and anyone who regularly spends a lot of time driving may sooner or later develop a chronic pain condition.

Chronic pain is a worldwide problem

The statistics on chronic pain are frightening. More than 20 per cent of people in Europe, including the UK, and 25 per cent of the American population have the condition. It is said that one in five Europeans has lost their job as a result, and 90 per cent of all those with the condition have not had their pain formally assessed. Chronic pain is not fully recognized and therefore is under treated and generally given a very low priority. An illustration of this is that many medical schools do not make the study of chronic pain a compulsory subject. I experienced the consequences of this when I was invited by a leading medical school to teach a section of the course on chronic pain – the programme was cancelled at the last minute because students failed to elect for the course of study. This happened in three consecutive years. Chronic pain is not a glamorous subject and it does not command big budgets within the health service.

Chronic pain in old age

In old age there can be no independence without fitness.

Neville Shone

The scale of the problem is even greater among the older generation, as the number of people in chronic pain is greatest in those aged over 55 years, until, by the age of 65, two-thirds are affected.

We live at a time when politicians, out of economic necessity, are extolling the virtues of extending the working life and raising the retirement age. It is true that life expectancy has increased. Officially, men in the UK can now expect to live to 80 and women to 83, with many surviving to 100. Are these people, many of whom are experiencing chronic pain, going to enjoy their remaining years or are they dreading the thought?

A number of research projects have highlighted pain as a significant yet neglected problem among old people, leading to multiple health problems. The research suggests there is a need for improved education, both for healthcare professionals and old people themselves, concerning attitudes to pain and ageing. There is considerable evidence to suggest that a significant proportion of old people with pain do not receive adequate pain management; this is not surprising, as very few people are actually referred to hospital for an assessment of their pain. A study was carried out at Nottingham University in 2002 on the management of pain within the local nursing home population (68 out of 121 nursing homes took part in a questionnaire survey.) The results showed that 69 per cent of these homes did not have a written policy regarding pain management and 75 per cent did not use a standardized pain assessment tool. Some 40 per cent of qualified staff and 85 per cent of care assistants had no specialist knowledge regarding the management of pain in this group of people. This was just a small study but I have no reason to believe that the situation is any different elsewhere in the country or that it has improved much, if at all, since 2002.

There seems to be a general acceptance by health professionals and older people themselves that pain is a side effect of old age and is something to be accepted. This fallacy has been allowed to go unchecked. Pain is not age-related and there is no reason why anyone with pain should be neglected. Everybody has colluded in ignoring the reality of the problem. Every citizen is entitled to equal treatment from the National Health Service (NHS), and this means providing a full consultant's assessment of chronic pain and a treatment plan that involves more than a prescription for painkillers. State provision has centred on providing basic physical care, such as warmth and shelter, and treating life-threatening illness, with little emphasis on preserving quality of life and preventing decline. Is something more needed, and is it right to expect the state to provide it?

How can those with chronic pain help themselves?

People with chronic pain, short on energy and stamina and being mainly on the wrong side of 55, are not in a position to fight their own cause in order to gain recognition from government or charities, let alone set up a nationwide organization to publicize their plight. Pain does not seem to attract backing from celebrities and this seems to be a prerequisite for opening doors to publicity and fund-raising.

There are some small local charities who do good work with individuals and at least one that distributes information on chronic pain and is represented on professional bodies concerned with pain. However, there is one charitable organization, Pain Association Scotland, which has been working in the field of chronic pain for over 20 years. The association has developed from a small group offering mutual support to an organization that has developed professional expertise in setting up and supporting groups in approximately 40 communities all over Scotland, including hospital settings, where it works in partnership with the medical profession. Because of the care taken over its development work it is now supported by medical organizations, voluntary bodies and local authorities. Its work might be said to represent an effective model for the establishment of self-help activity in the field of chronic pain. So successful has it been that it is now accepted as a preferred provider of chronic pain self-management services by the Scottish government. The work of the association is being studied by the Australian government, which is in the process of setting up its own chronic pain management services. Pain Association Scotland has a helpline (see Useful addresses at the end of the book) and is always willing to advise individuals and groups seeking help.

The national charity Arthritis Care also offers community-based pain management courses (see Useful addresses).

Self-help in pain management

I was fortunate that some months after the events recounted in the Prologue I was referred to Walton Hospital in Liverpool, where a pain management course had just started. I had a full assessment of my pain and was offered a place on a new course. This was the first such course to be established in Europe. For a full account of the provision of pain clinics and pain management courses, together with details of what to expect on a pain management course, see my book *Coping Successfully with Pain* published by Sheldon Press. The book also tracks my own progress and subsequent development in my attempt to rebuild my life.

Having spent some years working in an honorary capacity with the Walton Hospital team I began to develop my ideas for promoting pain management courses within the community and away from the white-coated hospital atmosphere. Having worked in the field for so long it is my belief that medical treatment by itself is only a small part of the solution to the problem. In the last 30 years it has become generally accepted that chronic pain needs a multi-faceted approach involving the talents of doctors, psychologists, physiotherapists, occupational therapists, acupuncturists and possibly psychotherapists and perhaps even more. There will always be a need for a hospital-based pain management service but in view of the numbers of potential patients and the demands on the service, something more is needed.

When I wrote *Coping Successfully with Pain* I had no idea that so many people would actually use the book to plan their own self-help programme, or that Pain Association Scotland would take up its message so wholeheartedly. I have received many letters from people with chronic pain, some of whom have been on two-year hospital waiting lists, saying that they no longer need to go on the hospital course because they have followed the ideas in the book and are now back in control of their lives and have resumed their careers. Several consultants in pain management have told me that they give copies of the book to patients when they know that they are likely to have to wait a very long time to get on a course.

Over the last 30 years the integrated approach to dealing with chronic pain has gradually become accepted. Initially, the idea that medication was not enough and needed to be supported by exercise, relaxation and behavioural therapies met with resistance, usually in the form of statements that funding bodies would need evidence that this approach worked. Most of the evidence, at that time, had been built up in the USA and for some reason was not enough on which to base a UK chronic pain management service. Thanks to the work of the pain management team at Walton Hospital, the research work of the Pain Foundation in Liverpool, the Pain Society and others, there is no longer any question about the value of this integrated approach.

However, there remains the problem of so many people with pain in the community and the increasing numbers approaching old age facing the prospect of living up to 40 years without help and with a deteriorating quality of life. An acquaintance of mine in his mid-50s, who has had pain for the last 20 years, asked his doctor for an assessment of his pain by a consultant. However, he was told that his pain history was too long and a consultation would be too late to be of any help. He continues with prescriptions for stronger painkillers, antidepressants, muscle relaxants and sleeping tablets. These make no impression whatsoever on his pain but his faith in the treatment has not diminished.

It is this overall situation that prompted me to tackle this project and make available the teaching material I have used when working directly with people in pain. Considering the numbers of people with chronic pain, few will have access to pain management courses. However, many can benefit from working alone, provided they are given some structure to follow. Many more can benefit from working together in groups. It may be that existing informal support groups can give a better service to those with chronic pain if the groups have a more formal structure and some guidance.

What is the approach of the book?

My background is in social work, psychotherapy, group work and education, and my experience in these fields has been added to my experience as someone who has lived with chronic pain for about

40 years. It is my belief that if any inroads are to be made into the problem of chronic pain then education should play a major part, both in treatment and prevention.

The approach of this book is therefore educational. The material is presented in the form of a course very similar to those I have led with chronic pain groups. The emphasis is on developing physical fitness systematically and progressively. Of course it is expected that over a period of time people will take responsibility for extending themselves physically, bearing in mind their limited capabilities. Even becoming marginally fitter should bring encouragement. Learning the skill of relaxation is crucial to the course, both as an essential element of pain relief and in order to combat stress. Information about pain and its consequences is included to take away any mystique and to lay the foundation for making changes in attitude and behaviour. If you feel in any way apprehensive about tackling the course then be assured.

How do I use the book?

If you are working on your own, work entirely at your own pace. You do not have to tackle the whole course at once. It is divided into six separate sessions. Ideally, each session should be completed on one day each week over a six-week period. The intervening days should be used to repeat the physical and relaxation exercises to become familiar with the routines. However, as long as you exercise every day and follow the breathing and relaxation programmes you may spread the rest of the course out as you wish.

I have tried to keep paragraphs short without losing too much information. Repetition is there for a purpose – repetition aids learning. I know that pain and the fatigue it brings places a limit on your capacity to read and assimilate long passages of text.

Working on your own can seem hard, especially if there is no one around to give you praise or feedback. The problem with working alone is that you have to be a good self-starter and be able to keep yourself motivated. I hope that the prospect of being able to manage your pain is enough to get you started and that the following pages will be enough to inspire you to keep motivated. Take frequent breaks as you go through the course and remember to reward yourself in some way as you complete each phase of the course. It may sound like hard work, and it is, but it is pleasurable and you should begin to see results very quickly.

Does it help to work in a group?

From an early age all our learning takes place within the context of one group or another, such as family, school, Scouts and Guides or football teams. Group influence is very powerful and has a profound effect on all our behaviour, good and bad. The literature concerned with therapy provides many examples of ways in which groups can be used to bring about beneficial change for individuals experiencing difficulties. Groups are a means of support and help. They involve people working together to improve facilities or share their resources of knowledge, skill and understanding. Group work is a skill available to all people, not only professionals. There is a richness of voluntary self-help activity relating to a wide range of community life. This richness helps to sustain many people and gives them pleasure and satisfaction and brings the rewards that come from sharing with others important aspects of their daily lives. The group is not just a background against which people perform – it is the actual instrument which enables them to grow and become self-sufficient.

The real strength of the group lies in the mutual support that people offer each other. It is not dependent on the special expertise of specific members or leaders. However, all self-help groups need a focus and the support of many people if they are to be successful. One of the reasons for bringing together a group of people who have a common problem is that they will all have tried to find a solution for coping with their problem. Some will have been more successful than others and some may feel totally defeated. In sharing ways in which they coped, or did not cope, each may learn something that will be of value and support as they experience the change that results from new learning. The group can create an environment where an appropriate level of trust can develop, and as people interact more easily with each other they may recognize that they are not as different, isolated or incompetent as they thought.

Learning in a group situation carries a great deal of conviction. There are two major advantages: (1) the recognition that others have coped with similar problems, and (2) the message seems to have more credibility and learning is more rapid when conveyed by a group of people who have first-hand experience. In modern parlance they have 'been there, done it, got the T-shirt'.

The professional's knowledge of chronic pain and its treatment may be profound but this knowledge is of a different quality from that of the people who live with the problem. The job of a leader is to enable the group members to tap into their collective knowledge and use it for the benefit of all. When people are overwhelmed by their problem, such as chronic pain, they lose sight of all those resources that have been gained over a lifetime. No matter how poor a person's ability to cope may have been in the past, experience in the group, combined with new knowledge and skills, may form the basis of developing better coping behaviour in the future.

Those who have had personal experience – and survived or improved their ability to cope – have much greater credibility. There are many examples of people being able to help each other when they come together with a common problem. Take, for example, Alcoholics Anonymous, who use common experience as a basis for change. Working on the problem in a group situation can do much to alleviate suffering. With the support of others who share the pain experience, it is often easier to take on new learning, change unhelpful behaviour and develop new coping skills. The emphasis is on working together to achieve a better quality of life. Services for people with chronic pain in the UK have been slow to develop in certain areas and it is hoped that this programme will go some ways towards reactivating physically, emotionally and spiritually those people who would otherwise remain neglected.

At the end of this book is an Appendix intended to give guidance to group leaders on how to organize and manage group sessions.

Session 1

This course is aimed at helping you to:

- reduce your level of pain so that you can regain control and mastery over your life and fill your days with thoughts and activities that do not include pain;
- become fitter;
- become more socially active;
- reduce levels of anxiety and depression;
- reduce intake of pain medication;
- plan ahead;
- develop new strategies for coping with your pain and setbacks;
- maintain all the improvements you make, experience a better quality of life and perhaps return to work.

These are the objectives I would like you to aim for. I know they are possible from my own experience and from the feedback I have had from the many people I have worked with over the years. Impartial research shows that for most people, following a course like this produces positive results and is far more effective than painkillers alone. All successful pain management schemes have something in common in that they teach forms of exercise and relaxation, which are the basis of most of the techniques you will learn in controlling your pain.

However, it is not entirely up to me to lay down aims and objectives for you. As a teacher I have the obligation to show you the way and demonstrate the techniques to enable you to succeed, but *you* have to make a commitment to work at the programme as outlined, at your own pace, and you have to engage daily, whether or not you have pain and no matter how bad you might feel. Imagine that you are an athlete preparing for the Olympic Games. Olympic athletes accept that to succeed they have to work, putting in time every day. It is difficult at first but it gets easier and the rewards are priceless.

I still remark to my wife after many years of working on exercise, relaxation and mental exercises: 'Do you know I couldn't do that six months ago?' as I reflect on some regained skill that I thought had been lost forever.

In our society, most of us have surrendered the responsibility for our health to the NHS, endowing it with magical powers to produce the right pill or form of treatment that will take away all our problems. So we are bound to be disappointed when the treatment does not work. We feel abandoned. Our trust has been shattered. This is the time we have to begin a process of learning that true healing comes from within, and that we need help to discover resources within ourselves that can help in this process. Sometimes on very bad days, when I have been tempted to curl up in a corner, I have remembered my training in pain management. I go back to basics and follow my programme of exercise and relaxation knowing that it will help me to recover sufficiently to go off and enjoy the rest of the day. So, now you can begin . . .

Activity 1
Be clear about your aims

This is your chance to establish what you would like to achieve for yourself as a result of following this course. Sometimes people start on a new venture without being clear about why they are doing it. Think carefully, and begin by stating what you would like to gain from the course and what you are aiming for. Now write it down. It will then be easier for you to assess the changes that are taking place in your condition as you progress through the various sections. If you are part of a group going through this course you will have the opportunity to share your aims with the others. If you are working independently make sure the people around you know what you are aiming for and invite their support. They may want to join in the various activities.

In general terms your aims will be consistent with the ones I have outlined, but of course everyone is different and you may have a specific goal that might seem impossible at this moment. I know that what helped me as I was going through the pain management course was the target I set myself of walking my daughter down the aisle three months later. In fact, establish for yourself a specific target and write it down. Pin it up on the wall where you can see it each day as a reminder. It does not have to be something outrageously ambitious such as a marathon.

Jim set himself an unrealistic target. He had been a very fit man taking part in lots of sports. He measured 'manliness' in terms of physical achievement. Now, and for two years previously, he needed two sticks to support him when out walking. He was 13 kg (2 stone) overweight and his breathing was laboured. His first target was to get back to refereeing a football match within a month of the course starting. He was building in failure, both for himself and the course leaders.

You need to aim for something manageable and realistic; otherwise you are in for a disappointment. Keep it simple, and when you achieve it you will find it easier to establish new goals and work towards them. For some people, just leaving the house and walking to the end of the street is an achievement.

Jane set herself the target of flying to the USA to visit her daughter after a five-year absence; I received a postcard from Jane just three months after the course had finished. She had started the course seemingly inseparable from her wheelchair and making demands that other people should fetch and carry for her.

Many people feel overwhelmed and helpless, as though nothing they try to help themselves will succeed. Every problem is too big. It is likely that such people will have a high degree of depression and will have some difficulty in specifying a goal to aim for. They may need help from a course leader or member of their family to formulate a very simple goal. So, if you recognize yourself here you should confide in someone close to you and ask them to help you set your target.

Topic A
Exercise is the key

No harm can come from movement

If you have had an injury or illness, healing will have taken place after three weeks or so. But although healing might have taken place you could still be experiencing pain. You may, as I once did, have a fear of movement, anxious that you might do more damage and increase your pain. You may prefer to find the most comfortable position you can and stay there for as long as possible; however, all the evidence points to the fact that no harm can come from movement. When you are active you feel better and your anxiety, stress and pain are reduced.

Unnecessary rest does not help

Pain has traditionally been treated on the assumption that it will ease if you rest. Rest will help in periods of acute illness or during recovery from injury or surgery. It is vital at these times to let the body heal itself. When we do not exercise, muscles waste, bones lose their mass and become brittle, the heart and lungs cease to function efficiently, blood flow is reduced and waste is not effectively eliminated. Balance is adversely affected and we begin to stumble and fall. This is particularly bad for anyone who is older or who already has a spinal condition such as spinal stenosis. If you have a chronic pain condition bed rest is *not* the answer. Even three days bed rest can decrease stamina by 25 per cent. The longer you remain inactive the harder it will be to regain strength. Unnecessary rest is no help to anyone with chronic pain.

Exercise helps you feel better

When you are sitting around brooding and anticipating trouble you do not feel good. You may feel depressed dwelling on all the bad things that have happened in the past and feeling sorry for yourself.

The exercises in this programme are gentle, involve no strain and their purpose is to retrain the body into increasingly normal movement. They will help you to increase mobility, develop flexibility and improve circulation to all parts of your body. As you develop a greater range of motion in your joints you will feel stronger and more able to cope with physical demands. If you follow the exercises in the programme, without setting targets that are too ambitious and not doing too much too soon, you will feel better, more positive and you will develop a greater sense of well-being and confidence. Your feeling of depression will ease.

Exercise produces chemical reactions in the body that have a direct effect on your pain and also serve to ease depression. Research indicates that half an hour of exercise three times a week can ease some forms of depression as effectively as drug treatment.

Know your limits

Always go gently, set manageable targets and do not strain. Remember, these exercises are designed particularly for people who have been inactive for a long time and may have fears about damaging themselves. It is essential to start slowly, setting realistic targets for each exercise. It is better to try to perform one repetition of each exercise than to use all your energy performing multiple repetitions of just a few. Your body is being retrained so it is important not to show off and exercise to the point of tiredness. Systematic, progressive exercise done frequently is better than exercising to the point of exhaustion once a week.

Get help if you need it

Before beginning any course of exercise take medical advice on whether it is suitable for you. If you are living alone and you have difficulty getting up and down from the floor without assistance then it is better to have someone to support you for these sessions.

Activity 2
Physical exercise

To get the greatest benefit from any exercise programme you should exercise regularly, at least three or four times a week. Ideally, exercise daily.

The exercises described below are progressive, which means that you start this programme with very simple exercises that involve little or no strain on muscles which have not been used for a long time.

Some of the exercises require you to use a ball. However, this is only essential in the first exercise, the back massage. Otherwise, you can substitute a scarf or a wooden spoon just to keep your hands in position.

As the programme continues you will be asked to add further exercises that may be more demanding. You do not have to repeat the same exercises each time; you can vary them to add interest. What is important is that you attempt to stretch and strengthen every part of your body. If you can, exercise in a group or with a friend. You will find it much more fun and you can encourage each other. The exercises throughout the programme include chair exercises which are suitable for older people, particularly those with disabilities or poor balance and for anyone who has trouble standing or getting down on the floor to exercise.

Start by sitting up straight with your bottom tucked into the back of the chair and your feet flat on the floor. Ideally, use a straight-backed dining chair or something similar.

Arm and shoulder stretch

This exercise works on the middle of your back, arms and shoulders. Interlace your fingers and turn your palms away from you. Stretch your arms in front of you at shoulder height, breathing in as you do so. Hold the breath for a count of five and as you breathe out slowly return your hands to your chest. Repeat five times.

This exercise can be done at any time of the day, standing or sitting. It can help relieve tension in back and shoulder muscles.

Back massage and mobility

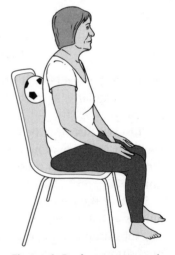

You will need a ball for this exercise. Place it behind you as you sit in your chair and lean against it, with your upper back holding the ball between you and the chair (see Figure 1). Move your torso from side to side and bend up and down to give yourself a massage. I find this exercise more satisfactory if I place the ball in different positions up my back. In this way it is possible to massage the whole of the back.

Figure 1 Back massage and mobility

Exercising the thigh muscles

Sit as illustrated in Figure 2, with the ball between your thighs. Squeeze your thighs gently together, breathing in as you do so. Hold the position and the breath for a count of five. Breathe out and release the tension. Repeat five times. You can use this exercise without a ball, using both fists clasped together between your thighs.

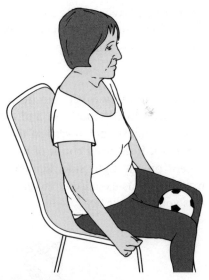

Figure 2 Exercising the thigh muscles

Ankle and foot exercise

Sit on your chair with knees bent. Hold on to the sides of the chair and extend both legs out in front of you. Now, bend the toes towards you and hold the position for a count of five (see Figure 3a). Lower your legs back down and repeat the movement eight to ten times. Next, extend both legs in front of you and point your toes away from you (see Figure 3b). Hold this position for a count of five. Repeat eight to ten times.

Now, raise and extend your right leg out in front of you and make circling movements with your foot, first in one direction and

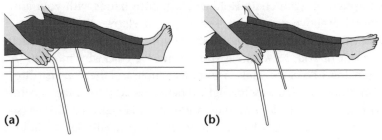

(a)   (b)

Figure 3 Ankle and foot exercise

then the other. When you have repeated this exercise five times, balance things up by doing the same with your left foot. This exercise can be done in bed before you get up.

Neck stretch

Sit upright in your chair and slowly tilt your head toward your left shoulder. Hold your head in this position and extend your right arm out to the side and slightly downward so that your hand is at waist level (see Figure 4). Hold for a count of five and then slowly repeat the movement on the right side. Remember to keep your torso upright throughout this exercise; it is very easy to lean your body to one side as you tilt your head.

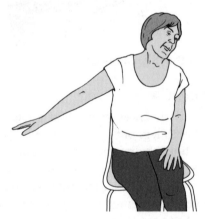

Figure 4 Neck stretch

Arm circles

Sit upright in your chair. Hold a ball in both hands with your arms extended above your head, keeping your elbows slightly bent. If you cannot extend your arms above your head then extend them in front of you. Now, circle your arms in a clockwise motion, the top being 12 o'clock. Make a complete circle and then reverse direction. Carry on this way for eight repetitions. Rest for a few seconds with arms lowered and then do another set of eight repetitions (see Figures 5a and 5b). A ball is not essential; instead you can hold a scarf or a wooden spoon.

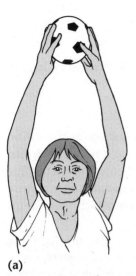
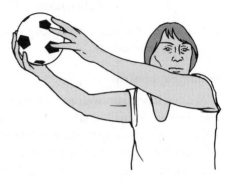

(a)   (b)

Figure 5 Arm circles

Elbow to knee

Sit upright in your chair. Extend
your right arm to the front and
slowly raise your left knee towards
your chest. At the same time bend
your elbow and bring it down to
meet your left knee. Repeat this
action eight to ten times and then
repeat on the other side, using your
left arm and right knee (see Figure
6). If you are feeling confident you
can try this exercise in a standing
position.

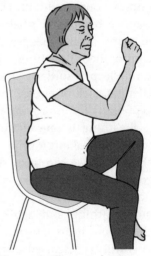

Have a chair or other support by
you in case you need help with your
balance.

Figure 6 Elbow to knee

Well done! Now it is time to have
a break.

Topic B
Relaxation – Breathing

When you achieve one simple goal you gain confidence and an impetus to build on your success.

Regaining control

When we have pain we can feel overwhelmed; it seems there is no way we can control what is happening to us and we feel helpless. This is very destructive. We are shaken to the core and we become anxious. We may even go into a downward spiral, and when we reach the bottom it is a dark, lonely place from which there seems to be no way back.

It is important to find a way to get back in control. Regaining control of our lives when we seem to have lost it completely may seem impossible. Having control over our lives involves exercising the ability to make choices. When we have pain and feel helpless there seems to be little scope for us to make *any* choices that will improve our condition. Despite this we can choose to change the way we breathe. A small change, indeed, but one that can lead to many bigger changes. Breathing is the key to getting back in control. Poor breathing is a key factor in asthma, high blood pressure, sleep disorders, stress, anxiety, headaches, shoulder pain, allergies, lack of energy and other illnesses. Breathing is the best-kept secret for improving your health.

Breathing is one of those functions that is partly under conscious control but for the most part continues without us thinking about it. If we can bring our breathing under control, and it feels good, what is to say we cannot take control of other bodily functions? Evidence and personal experience show that we can control our breathing and achieve a state of relaxation. We can also change our heart rate and reduce blood pressure – and pain levels. This will be discussed further when we focus on biofeedback and self-hypnosis.

These unconscious processes are directly influenced by the way we breathe. We just need to learn how to breathe properly. Once you have learned this method you will find it helps to control your pain, reduce anxiety, ease depression, improve sleep, lower blood pressure and help your body eliminate impurities. In fact, every aspect of your health will benefit.

Shallow breathing

People in pain who are anxious or tense breathe in a shallow way, high in the chest, increasing tension in all parts of the body. You no doubt experience this yourself. You feel tightness in the chest and throat and may even experience panic attacks, which make you sweat and struggle with your breathing.

Babies breathe correctly, completely relaxed and with the breath moving in and out on the diaphragm or tummy area. As we grow older we tend to lose this rhythmic, relaxing way of breathing. We experience fear, anxiety and pain. We become tense and the rhythm is upset.

If you have pain your situation can be made worse, as incorrect breathing creates tense muscles and reduces the oxygen supply to the rest of the body. This produces a vicious circle of pain–tension–pain–anxiety and fear–more tension–more pain–increased anxiety and fear–increased pain . . . People with pain and tension often have a disturbed sleep pattern, resulting in exhaustion and low energy levels. Exhausted, tense bodies are strong candidates for more pain and minds will be attacked by streams of negative thoughts and images. The quickest way to release this tension is to relearn how to breathe properly.

Diaphragmatic breathing

Correct diaphragmatic breathing helps break this vicious circle by releasing tension, reducing anxiety and fear and, more importantly, controlling pain. Many people who learn this technique have told me how effective it is as a therapeutic aid and, for them, has been enough to help them live full lives without the need for medication.

Initially, you will need to set aside times to practise the breathing technique. Eventually, it will become second nature, automatic and unconscious. You will recognize those situations that upset your breathing rhythm and regain your composure through breathing. Apart from pain episodes, the most common life events that upset breathing are arguments, waiting on the telephone while the recorded voice at the other end goes through a list of options, when you feel your computer has a life of its own and you are ready to throw it through the window and when your children test your patience . . . You will no doubt be able to add a few more.

Diaphragmatic breathing is a skill you once had but may have forgotten over your lifetime. I will show you how to regain this skill, which is at the heart of meditation programmes, hypno-therapy, yoga, t'ai chi and the martial arts. Once you have mastered this technique you will be able to use it whenever you want and, with practice, it will become second nature.

How to practise diaphragmatic breathing

Be comfortable

Prepare by getting ready a blanket or duvet and two pillows, one for your head and one for under your knees. When you relax com-pletely the body loses heat, so it is wise to cover yourself. Lower the light level. You do not want to be distracted by the sun or a lamp shining in your eyes. Find a comfortable place to lie flat on the floor, allowing enough space to stretch your arms out to the side without touching anything. Lie down on your back, legs straight in front or with knees bent, and feet flat on the floor. It is not essential to lie down but it helps while you are learning.

If you find it difficult to get down on the floor then sit comfort-ably in a chair in a balanced position, with your bottom well back into the seat, legs uncrossed and hands resting gently on your thighs.

Become aware of your breathing

Focus your attention on your diaphragm, just below your ribcage, and gently rest your hands at that point, fingertips just touching. This area will rise and fall in rhythm with your breathing. Imagine you have a balloon under your fingers and on the in breath feel the balloon inflating; as it does so your fingertips will part. As you breathe out they will come back together and you will feel your balloon deflate. You may find this strange at first because it seems to be the opposite of the way you normally breathe but practice will soon make it feel normal. Continue breathing into the diaphragm for ten complete breaths.

Resist the temptation to puff out your chest and lift your shoulders. This method of breathing has historically been the method taught in old-style PE lessons and military training: 'Head up, chest out, shoulders back!' This style of breathing leads to tension in the head, neck, shoulders and back.

Once you are comfortable with this new method of breathing then slow your breathing down and allow your breath to become deeper. Think about the balloon inflating to fill the area around your ribs. Breathe in this way for a minute or two. Now, begin to count your breaths in and out. In to a count of four and out to a count of five. With practice you will find that you can do this steadily and without effort. You are in control of the breathing process.

When you practice this on other occasions, try increasing the length of the breaths, for example in for a count of six and out for a count of eight. It is the control and length of the out breath that is most important.

There is no rush in this exercise. Take as long as you like and you will probably find you will achieve a level of comfort and relaxation you have not experienced for a long time. Enjoy it.

Practice this method of relaxation when settling down to sleep. You will find it helps.

Monitor your breathing

Learn to monitor your breathing throughout the day. The rhythm of your breathing changes according to whatever you are doing, and from time to time you may find that your breathing is high in your chest and there is tightness in your chest and shoulders. These changes are likely to happen unconsciously, when you are talking, thinking, driving, worrying, watching an exciting TV programme, listening to someone else's tale of woe, or when you are emotionally or sexually aroused. If you monitor your breathing constantly it is possible to keep one small part of your mind focused on your breathing, so that you become aware of any changes instantly and can correct your breathing pattern. As your skill develops you will notice improvements in the way you feel, the way you relate to other people and the way you cope with stressful situations. The increased oxygen in your blood will make you feel brighter and more energetic, and other people will notice the changes – maybe even before you do. I remember people remarking to me shortly after I started the pain management programme how my face had changed. I no longer looked so haggard.

Let go of anxious thoughts

If you are not part of a group but are learning this skill by yourself, and are beginning to relax after long periods of tension or anxiety, it is quite possible that your mind will focus on anxious thoughts and feelings of anger and resentment about your situation or other people. Later on I will deal more fully with this topic but, for the time being, remember this is your quiet time and just let any thoughts drift through your mind. Do not hold on to them. Let them go. They are not important.

Group leaders

If you are a group leader, it is useful to ask each person for some feedback about their experience. Some can be quite upset or even disappointed if they have not achieved their goal. In my experience, many people embark on this beginner's session with the expectation that all their pain will be miraculously removed. Clarify with them exactly what it was they expected to happen and stress the importance of continuing to practise relaxation as a foundation to build on. It is the process of practising that is important at this stage. Even though most people find things difficult at the start, eventually they will develop the appropriate breathing rhythm.

Activity 3
Some questions about your pain

When I am working with a group I always take the opportunity in the first meeting to ask each person to talk about their pain and how it affects them. It helps to develop some kind of perspective on the whole experience of pain, so I provide them with a framework to present their thoughts to the rest of the group. If you are working alone you may like to think about the following questions and perhaps even write some notes for your own benefit. As you progress you might like to look back at them and see the point at which you started your journey back into health.

Writing things down may be easier, as some people find it difficult to talk about themselves and their problems. It may be that people with pain problems do not have the opportunity to talk things over with others and they may have protected family and friends from knowing very much about the full extent of their problems and fears. They may, instead, have found many non-verbal ways of communicating their difficulties or have expected people to be mind readers. Whatever you write down can be for your eyes only so you can be totally honest. In a group, sharing things verbally still leaves you in control and you can share as much or as little as you like, but generally I find that people welcome the opportunity to talk. After all, everyone is working towards a common goal.

- How long have you had your pain?
- Have you been told that it is related to some illness, injury or operation?
- What parts of your body are affected?
- What impact has it had on your life in general; on your work, relationships and social activities?

Activity 4
Progressive Muscle Relaxation

It is important to develop an awareness of when you are tense and when you are relaxed.

What is Progressive Muscle Relaxation?

At times, you may think you are relaxed but your muscles can still be holding on to tension. Many people think relaxation means lounging on the sofa watching TV or sitting over a pint in the pub. This is not the case!

Progressive Muscle Relaxation helps you to reduce the *resting tension* in your muscles by tensing and then relaxing individual muscle groups in various parts of the body. As a result, you become increasingly aware of areas that may be holding tension and, with practice, you will be able to distinguish between states of tension and relaxation. Once you have reached that stage you are well on the way to controlling your pain or preventing it developing. The technique has been shown to be successful in treating and preventing stress-related conditions such as high blood pressure, tension headaches and pain. In my own work with clients I have used it successfully in treating people with anxiety states as well as those with painful conditions. It was developed early in the twentieth century by the American physiologist Edward Jacobson, who maintained that anxiety resulted in muscle tension and that reducing this tension would allow the body's stress response to diminish.

When we have pain we tend to tense other parts of our body to compensate. This tension can become a permanent feature of our lives, if we allow it, and as a result many people experience general-ized pain that does not seem to be focused in one particular spot. As a result the whole body is sore and subject to spasm. I often talk to people I am working with about the importance of 'putting the pain back in its rightful place'. For example, you might start off with back pain and, over time, experience pain throughout your body. When this happens you can feel as though your condition has deteriorated or that you have developed cancer or some other potentially fatal condition. We fear the worst as our anxiety grows. The result may be more visits to the doctor, increasing medication and becoming more isolated, anxious and depressed. Learning the skill of Progressive Muscle Relaxation can directly help us to relieve the body of its disabling tensions.

A study in 2004, which took place in the Purdue School of Nursing in Indiana, showed that Progressive Muscle Relaxation achieved significant reductions in pain and mobility problems for the osteoarthritis patients taking part. A big advantage of practising Progressive Muscle Relaxation is that it can be carried out any-where, without the need of any special equipment. All you need to do is to sit or lie down in a comfortable position and focus on the various muscle groups in turn.

It is such a powerful method of relaxation that you may find that it is the only skill you need to help you cope with your pain, and no matter how many setbacks you have it will work every time. For some people it is as though they are experiencing full and deep relaxation for the first time.

As an aid, I have recorded the following Progressive Muscle Relaxation sequence on CD in the form of a relaxation programme. This can be ordered for a nominal charge from Pain Association Scotland, who benefit from the sale of this and other CDs that I have recorded. Details are given at the end of the book under 'Useful addresses'.

Instructions for Progressive Muscle Relaxation

1   Sit in a fully supported position on a chair or lie down on your back on the floor. If lying down, cover yourself with a blanket or duvet. Become aware of your breathing for a minute or two. Experience the in breath flowing into the diaphragm and allow your out breath to flow easily and comfortably, without any pause between the in and out breaths.

2   When your breathing is steady and comfortable, focus your attention on your arms. Lift them slightly, extend them and clench your fists as hard as you can and hold your breath to a count of five. Let the tension go, breathing out as you do so and let the arms fall back into the resting position. Repeat this exercise three times. Then take note of the way your muscles feel now that they are relaxed. Feel the warmth of the increased blood flow into your arms, hands and fingers.

3   Take a deep breath and hold it while raising your shoulders towards your ears, at the same time pulling your head down towards your shoulders. Hold the breath and the tension for a count of five, then release the breath and the tension and allow the shoulders to relax completely. Repeat three times.

4   Take a deep breath into the chest and hold it for a count of five while tensing the muscles in the chest area. Then, let go of the breath and the tension, allowing all the muscles to relax completely. Repeat three times.

Take a moment to rest and breathe comfortably into your diaphragm for several moments. Now, in your own time, carry on with the next exercise.

5   If you are lying down, bend your knees slightly and tighten the muscles around your abdomen and pelvic area. Breathe in, hold

the breath and the tension for a count of five and then let go of the breath and the tension. Repeat three times.

This is a good point to pause and take note of what is happening in your body. You should be aware of an increased blood flow and a feeling of warmth beginning to spread through your body. Check your breathing again. Is it calm and steady? As you continue with these exercises make sure you breathe out completely as you let go of the tension.

6   Tighten the muscles of your buttocks as hard as you can. Take a deep breath and hold the tension and the breath for a count of five. Let go of the tension and the breath, allowing the muscles to relax completely. Repeat three times.

7   Tighten the muscles of the thighs as hard as you can. Take a deep breath; hold the tension and the breath for a count of five. Let go of the tension and the breath, letting the muscles relax completely. Repeat three times.

8   With your feet together and legs stretched out in front of you, tighten the muscles of your feet and calves by pointing your toes away from you as hard as you can. Take a deep breath; hold the tension and the breath for a count of five. Now, let go of the tension and the breath, allowing the muscles to relax completely. Repeat three times.

9   With feet together and legs stretched out in front of you, tighten the muscles of your feet and calves by pointing your toes towards you as far as you can. Take a deep breath; hold the tension and the breath for a count of five. Now, let go of the tension and the breath, allowing the muscles to relax completely. Repeat three times.

Now, rest quietly for a few moments. Restore your breathing into your diaphragm and experience the feeling of complete relaxation throughout your whole body.

10 This final exercise is particularly good for people with head, face and neck pains. Try not to be self-conscious about this one. Set out to enjoy it; if you feel like laughing, go ahead, because laughter helps to reduce tension better than any other exercise. Start by tightening the muscles around the jaw and neck area.

At the same time stretch the mouth into a grinning expression, stick out your tongue as far as you can, screw up your eyes, take a deep breath, hold the tension and count to five. Then let go of the tension and the breath and relax completely. Repeat three times.

11 The next part of this exercise requires you to open your eyes wide and look up to the ceiling. At the same time open your mouth wide and allow your jaw to drop. Now, stick out your tongue, take a deep breath and hold the position for a count of five. Then let go of the breath, close the mouth and eyes and . . . relax completely. Continue to lie or sit in this relaxed position for as long as you wish, breathing steadily into the diaphragm.

Topic C
Track your progress with a diary

For your own guidance keep a daily diary. Unless you do you will only have a vague idea of your progress. A diary will show you how you are progressing as you follow this course. Do not think of it as a chore but as a contribution to your progress towards taking control of your life again. Below are some of the things you should be recording.

- Do you have less pain?
- Are you having fewer episodes of pain?
- Do you recover from flare-ups more quickly?
- Are you getting more involved with other people?
- Do you enjoy life more?
- Are you doing new things?
- Are you sleeping better?
- How is your libido?
- Are you using less medication?
- Are you able to stand, sit or walk for longer periods?
- Are jobs in the home less arduous?

Keeping a diary will help to pinpoint the particular day when things begin to improve. It may also help you to see what part of the programme is particularly helpful for you. Keep your diary private, for your eyes only, and only you will know if you skip your exercise and go back to your old habits.

Each day, record how you spend your time. Note how long you spend lying in bed or on a sofa, how far you walk and for how long, how many exercises and repetitions you complete. From my experience if you can spend less time sitting or reclining and more time moving about you are more likely to have less pain and feel better.

In particular, make a note of how you find the exercises. Are they getting easier? Is your recovery time getting shorter? Record how difficult you find the breathing and relaxation exercises and, as you progress, note the benefits.

Take a note of your pain level – ideally each hour during the day – but if this is not possible then record it three times a day, morning, afternoon and evening. Give your pain level a score from 1 to 10; the higher the score, the more severe the pain. Pay attention to the time each pain episode lasts. You may have peaks at certain times, which can be related to some things you are doing, or are not doing, or to spending too much time on one activity. See if your pain is as bad when you are inactive as it is when you are busy. Remember, no one feels pain all the time or feels the same intensity of pain from one hour to the next.

If you are on medication make a point of noting when and how much you take, and whether the medication has a direct influence on your pain or is merely making you sleepy or too drowsy to care. Are you taking prescribed medication or are you buying over-the-counter tablets – or maybe a mix of both? You may even put your trust in street drugs (remember, there is no way to know how much to take and, of course, there is no quality control so street drugs could be dangerous, especially if you mix them with other medication or alcohol). Note what side effects you experience; for example, constipation, indigestion, weight gain or even temporary oblivion.

Finally, make a note of all the positive things in your life each day. It may be that you have enjoyed a particular meal, had a visit from your grandchildren or enjoyed a good gossip with an old friend.

Take a week to absorb the information in this session and practise daily both the physical and relaxation exercises. Establish your diary and think very clearly about your commitment to making real changes. Do not be impatient with yourself. You have probably taken many years to develop your pain problem and it will take time to regain control over your life; but it will happen.

You have now reached the end of your first session and it is time to wind down from the hard work of the day and reflect on what you have learned. At this stage it is worth thinking about setting a target to achieve before the next session. Set yourself the target of completing all the physical, breathing and relaxation exercises every day. You may want to do more than that. I remember my first target was to sit through an entire meal with the family without getting up from the table. By the end of the first week I had achieved my target.

Session 2

This session will continue the pattern of the first, focusing on exercises to help you strengthen and stretch your muscles so that you have more flexibility and at the same time helping to reduce some of the tension in your body. The exercises in this session are also designed to improve your balance and posture and, of course, make you feel good. Now you have got the hang of diaphragmatic breathing, this session will take you further with your breathing and relaxation techniques and help you to focus on the more positive aspects of living.

The following topics will be explored: Beginning to think and behave in a positive way and Your food, your pain.

Activity 5
Physical exercise

Complete the exercises outlined in Session 1, performing as many repetitions as you are able without feeling any discomfort. You should now be well warmed up and ready to extend your range of physical activity. These additional exercises will offer new challenges and introduce some variety into your daily routine.

Side stretch

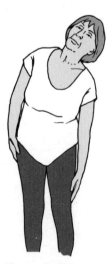

Stand with your feet slightly apart and your arms by your side. Take a breath in, and as you breathe out lean your trunk over to your left side, sliding your left hand down towards your knee (see Figure 7). Do not allow your body to lean forward. Hold the position for a count of five before slowly returning to the upright position. Repeat this movement to the left three times and then do the same exercise to your right side. Do not be tempted

Figure 7 Side stretch

to over-stretch. As you become more accustomed to this movement you may wish to make the exercise stronger by stretching the opposite arm towards your ear as you lean to the side.

Inner thigh stretch

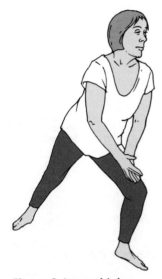

Stand with your legs apart, in line with your shoulders. Now, swivel your left foot to the left and face in that direction. Breathe in, and as you breathe out bend your left knee and place both hands on the knee. Breathing in, gently come into the upright position. Repeat this movement three times, remembering that the breathing is important. You will feel the stretch on the inside thigh of the straight leg (see Figure 8). Continue by bending the right knee and repeat three times. Alternatively, if your balance is good, you can raise your arms out to the side and do the bend in that position.

Figure 8 Inner thigh stretch

Balancing

Stand upright, facing forward, with the feet about 23 cm (9 inches) apart. Take a breath in, and keeping your legs straight, slowly raise your right foot a little way out to the side, and hold this position for as long as you can. Then, on an out breath, gently lower your foot to the floor. Repeat three times. Continue with the exercise using the left leg. If you need help to balance, rest your hand on the back of a chair to do this exercise (see Figure 9 overleaf).

Holding on to your chair, stand up straight facing forward, with feet about 23 cm (9 inches) apart. Breathe in and slowly raise your right foot to rest on the inner side of your left knee (see Figure 10 overleaf). If you cannot reach your knee just place it as high as you can. Hold the position for a count of five; then, on the out breath, lower the foot to the floor. Repeat three times, then do the exercise using the other leg and repeat three times.

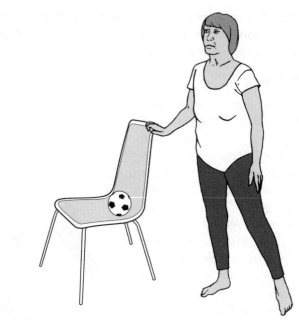

Figure 9 Balancing

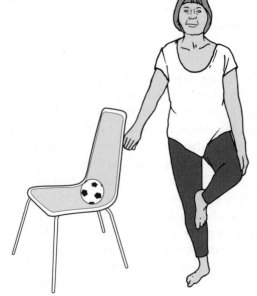

Figure 10 Balancing

Knee bends

This exercise is to help maintain the ability to climb steps. Stand with your feet apart and your back against a smooth door. Breathe in, and on the out breath slide your back down the door as far as you can, at the same time bending your knees (see Figure 11). Now breathe in and slowly slide your back up into the standing position.

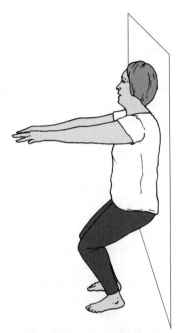

Activity 6
Relaxation

Prepare for relaxation under your duvet or blanket, or you may like to try this activity sitting on a chair. By the end of the course you should be able

Figure 11 Knee bends

to relax whether sitting or lying down. From my own experience, most people enjoy relaxing in the lying down position but by the end of this session there is another activity that will involve relaxing in the standing position.

Now, continue by going through the Progressive Muscle Relaxation sequence outlined in Session 1. By now you should be well practised at this. When you have completed the sequence, remain in your relaxed position while I take you through a relaxation session that involves focusing on positive memories.

If you are not part of a group it would be helpful to record the following passage or get someone close to read it out to you. Take care to speak slowly, and pause for several seconds where the dots appear. Where there are more dots then make the pause longer.

Continue your breathing and allow it to become slower . . . . and deeper . . . and remember . . . . . that this is your special time . . . . and in this special time nothing or no one should be allowed to intrude . . . .

In your own home you can set aside not only a special time but a special place away from normal domestic activities and family demands. In my own experience it took some time for my family to accept that when I closed my bedroom door for relaxation I was not 'on call'.

When we relax in this way we often find that thoughts enter into our minds without bidding . . . . . Often, these thoughts can disturb our relaxation . . . . increasing our heart rate, creating tension . . . . . This is not helpful. It is important that any thoughts that happen like this are acknowledged and then let go. Learn the importance of only allowing thoughts to enter your mind at your bidding . . . . Learn to say no, quite firmly, to any other thoughts that try to creep in . . . . To help you in this process, focus on a word such as 'calm' or 'quiet' or a sound such as 'Uuuu . . . mmmm', which you can repeat to yourself when you find your mind wandering . . . . It seems now to be generally accepted that when we think of happy times, enjoyable times . . . . that we feel good . . . . . . so this is an opportunity to allow your mind to focus on a memory . . . . a pleasant memory . . . . Pleasant memories recalled have a magical property . . . . All the feelings of pleasure and happiness you experienced, perhaps even many years ago . . . . return just as they were and have a profound effect . . . . on the way you feel now . . . . There are many times in your life when you have experienced real pleasure and happiness . . . . and as your relaxation deepens . . .memories from the past . . . . pleasant memories . . . . can resurface and you can feel so much better . . . . *At this point pause for at least one minute.*

Take some time to experience to the full that pleasant memory . . . . See it in full colour . . . . hear the sounds associated with it . . . . perhaps even feel aspects of that memory . . . . such as the warmth of the sun . . . . sand under your feet . . . . As you breathe in . . . . remember the smells associated with that memory . . . . Of course you do not have to be in a state of deep relaxation to recall pleasant memories . . . . it is possible to recall such memories at any time . . . . and these will work very effectively in triggering good, positive feelings . . . . and you can feel very comfortable . . . . . any time you like . . . . Like you, I have a whole repertoire of good memories and I call on them frequently . . . . Immediately, I feel my mood lifting and my pain fades . . . . One of my favourite memories, which gives me an instant lift . . . . is to take myself back to a time on holiday in Wales many years ago . . . . I was sitting on a river bank watching sand martins skimming over the river and seeing the sunlight sparkling on the surface of the water . . . . I only need to spend an instant in that memory and I feel better . . . . Your mind is very powerful and you have the capacity to use it to help you at any time . . . . Continue to enjoy your special time.

When you are ready . . . . . . become aware of your surroundings and slowly open your eyes and begin to move your fingers and toes and, in your own time, stand up feeling refreshed.

Topic D
Beginning to think and behave in a positive way

I hope by now that you are beginning to feel the benefit of your relaxation sessions, and that you are finding it easier each time you do them. This is good preparation for moving on towards thinking and behaving *positively*. In the first session you were asked to focus on some of the negative aspects of pain; now it is time to forget those negative thoughts and feelings – to put them behind you as you begin to focus on the good things that are happening to you now and will happen in the future. As you do this, the negative, bad experiences will be put into perspective. No one gains anything by dwelling on the negative aspects of the pain experience any longer than is necessary.

When we have bad experiences they seem to dominate our thinking, to a point when we believe that nothing good ever happened in our lives. In fact, if we sit down and coolly take stock, we will see that the greatest part of our experience has been positive. It is time to find ways of developing the habit of getting back in touch with these positive aspects. When I am working with a group I start this process of developing positive thinking by asking everyone in turn: 'What was the nicest thing that happened to you last week?' It is not a question we are normally asked and some people find it difficult to review everything that has happened and find a pleasurable experience. You might like to try this for yourself. 'What was the nicest thing that happened to you last week?'

A few words of caution: many people find that they can make a positive statement about something that happened in the past week, but then negate that positive statement by adding the dreaded word 'but'. For example, I went to the zoo with my grandchildren. We had a marvellous day but the pain next day was terrible. How easy it is to sabotage the experience of good feelings with one little word. It is interesting that, in the group situation, people quickly modified their statements when one person was challenged about turning a positive statement into a negative one.

It is important that you should separate out things that you do from the experience of pain, otherwise you become conditioned to expect that pain automatically follows activity, even enjoyable activity. This can become an excuse for not joining in social activities. Learn to enjoy the moment and do not anticipate pain.

Homework for the week

During the coming week record all the good things that happen to you and make a habit of talking about them with friends and family. Take care! Remember the evil 'but' word. Spend at least one day making only positive statements – about the weather, friends, politics. Talk about every experience only in positive terms; do not complain, and avoid criticism of everything and everybody. If you cannot, then change the subject. It will not be easy, but see how you get on. Think about whether the exercise changes the way you feel.

This section will be continued in Session 4, Topic H.

Activity 7
Exercise leading into relaxation

This is an exercise that has been very successful, both for me and for group members. During the last few years I have worked with groups of people of various nationalities who have been overwintering in Spain. Only a few understood English so it was important to find a way to communicate using very few and simple words. I found that this particular exercise worked for most people as I was able to physically demonstrate the movements and to build on them in each succeeding session.

Those of you who have experience of yoga may recognize similarities between the following exercise and your yoga practice. This is a complete physical workout and a real tension buster.

Many people who have pain, arthritis or other disabilities develop tell-tale signs in their body, by tilting to the left or right, or perhaps stooping. This tendency to get out of balance happens to everyone as they get older. You may have noticed that a person who has for many years carried a shoulder bag or briefcase has one shoulder noticeably higher than the other. Someone using a walking stick for support may develop tension on one side of the body and lean to one side as a result. People with pain, as you know, develop different ways of guarding themselves against the pain. This often means tensing muscles and, over a long period, the way you stand, sit or walk is altered in such a way that you find it difficult to maintain a vertical position. The following exercises are designed to help you to get your body back into balance.

In order to feel adjustments in your position it is better to do this exercise without shoes. Beware – woolly socks on a slippery floor are not a good idea; better to have bare feet or find a rubber mat to stand on.

1   Find space that allows you to extend your arms sideways without touching anyone or anything else.
2   Stand with your feet slightly apart (about 23 cm; 9 inches) and pointing straight ahead. If you are unsure about your balance then you may prefer to have a chair at your side for support.
3   Standing in this way may feel unnatural if you have adopted a splayed stance for comfort or if you are normally a bit pigeon-toed. It may also feel strange if your body has been out of balance for some time. Take a few moments to get used to this position. As your body adjusts to find a point of balance you may find yourself swaying. Just allow it to happen and do not worry about it. If at any time during this exercise you feel uncomfortable or distressed, sit down for a few moments until you can start again.

4 Fix your eyes at a point on the wall directly in front of you and try not to be distracted by movement or sounds around you.

5 Continue to stand in this way, with your arms hanging by your side, and draw yourself up to your full height. Feel as if you have a cord coming out of the top of your head, like a puppet. Your head should not tilt backwards or forwards. Check that your chin is parallel to the floor. Hold your head high and feel the cord pulling you up.

6 Now, relax and drop your shoulders.

7 Direct your breathing into your diaphragm and breathe through the nostrils to a count of 1 . . . 2 . . . 3 . . . 4 . . . in and 1 . . . 2 . . . 3 . . . 4 . . . out. Do not hold your breath after the in breath but make a smooth transition to the out breath. After ten full breaths just breathe normally, but still into the diaphragm.

8 Now, keeping the breathing to a four in and four out count, raise the arms out and up to shoulder level on the in breath and back down to the sides on the out breath. It is important to have the arms and the breathing synchronized. Remember the smooth transition from the in breath to the out breath. Repeat this movement ten times. When your arms are lowered to your sides they should be relaxed, with the hands and fingers hanging loose. Be conscious of your in breath gently lifting your arms away from your sides. You do not have to push them up. There should be no tension whatsoever in your body as you continue this exercise.

9 You may wish to move your feet around, bend your knees, shake your arms and hands and shrug your shoulders before moving on to the next part of the exercise.

10 Return to the balanced standing position and breathe in to a count of four and raise the arms to shoulder level, keeping the breathing and movement synchronized. This time breathe out to a count of eight, slowly lowering the arms to the sides in time with the breath. Repeat three times.

You will probably find that this is enough for the first time. In subsequent sessions we will develop this exercise to build up a programme that will exercise all parts of the body; as a result you will be stronger and more flexible, with a greater sense of balance. This is a sure way to get rid of tension in your muscles, improve blood flow throughout your body and, of course, reduce your pain levels.

Topic E
Some lifestyle considerations – Your food, your pain

Pain leads to weight gain

You may have found that you have put on a lot of weight since your activity level has reduced as a result of your illness or pain. I know that I did. Carrying extra weight is not helpful for anyone with a pain problem or with a condition that affects the joints, so you owe it to yourself to lighten the load.

When you are fully active you may be able to eat whenever and whatever you fancy, without making any appreciable difference to your weight. When you are less mobile your food intake matters. If you do not move about much you do not burn off the calories, and any surplus food goes to fat. Also, as you get older your metabolism slows down and you do not need so much food. Unfortunately, the message does not get through to your appetite and you tend to eat until that appetite is satisfied.

You may be on medication where weight gain is a side effect. If this is so, seek medical advice. It is important that you discuss any worries about your weight with your medical advisers or dietician, as being overweight can lead to further health problems.

Controlling your appetite

As you are beginning to learn ways of making changes that directly improve your pain, this is a good time to think about taking control of what you eat. You should by now see that you are able to control tension in your muscles and achieve relaxation, and that this is making some difference to you. Now, you can also begin to think about controlling your appetite and not allow your appetite to control you. I am not saying it is easy but it can be done.

May I tell you how I tackled it? Within a very short time of becoming ill I could not fasten my belt and felt very bloated. For some time I did nothing about it as I was more concerned about my pain. My family were concerned for my general health and were worried about the rate at which I was expanding. As I began to become more skilful at controlling my pain I had more energy and was able to focus more on the state of my body. The first step was to reduce the amount of food I ate by changing from a large dinner plate to a much smaller plate and replacing my favourite mug with a dainty china teacup. Gradually, I was able to move to having a substantial lunch, cut out snacks and foods like biscuits and crisps and just have a small meal such as egg on toast at about 6.00 p.m. and then nothing more until the next morning. Without doing anything else I began slowly to lose weight.

As time went on, and I got more interested in the question of nutrition, I took a serious look at what went into a meal. Fortunately, as a family, we all enjoy home-cooked food and very rarely buy ready-cooked meals, so it was possible to make changes. This is a big subject and a full account of these changes and the reasons for them are given in *The Chronic Pain Diet Book* published by Sheldon Press, which was the result of 15 years of research. In the meantime, you will find it helpful to increase your fruit and vegetable intake (but not potatoes) and reduce the amount of meat and animal fats you eat. Steam or grill food rather than fry it and if you find the taste is a bit bland experiment with herbs and spices.

Foods can increase inflammation

Food has a direct bearing on inflammation and, therefore, pain levels. I am unable to take painkillers and anti-inflammatory drugs based on aspirin, and therefore must use food to help me control inflammation and pain. Inflammation increases if the diet includes animal fats such as those found in red meat, dairy products and saturated cooking oils. Many people who have a pain problem or arthritis are also food sensitive. Their sensitivity may have a direct effect on their pain. It can also produce inflammation and swelling in the digestive tract, which limits the ability of the digestive system to digest food completely. If you are unaware that you have a food sensitivity then continued use of that food will further compromise the digestive tract, causing even more inflammation around the joints and, of course, exacerbating pain problems.

Many health problems are inflammatory, which means part of the body such as a muscle or a joint, the gut or the respiratory tract is inflamed. It is a sign that the body is over-reacting to something.

Of course, you may be taking anti-inflammatory drugs as part of your treatment and it would be unwise to stop these without a full discussion with your medical adviser. However, you need to be aware that the drugs may be masking an underlying sensitivity problem.

Apart from food sensitivity it may be that your diet is completely inappropriate. Perhaps I ought to explain a little further about an inappropriate diet. I have already mentioned animal products. Other things to avoid are sugar, sugary drinks, alcohol and processed foods. Processed foods in particular can contain large amounts of salt and sugar and chemicals designed to improved taste, colour and shelf life but they can have the effect of making an inflammation problem worse. In addition, high levels of sugar and salt are not helpful to someone fighting weight gain, water retention and an inflammation problem.

Alcohol is high in calories and may have an inflammatory effect on the body and can also lead to weight gain. Another factor about alcohol that you need to take into account is that although it may appear to relieve your pain temporarily, there is always a 'kick-back' effect and your pain levels can increase rapidly. I have known a number of people with pain problems who have tried 'alcohol therapy', only to find its long-term effects do a great deal of damage to their health.

Foods that can help

My solution to the problem of reducing pain and inflammation without drugs, in addition to exercise and relaxation, is a diet rich in vegetables and oily fish such as salmon, herring, sardines and mackerel. These help the body produce a number of anti-inflammatory compounds.

Arrowroot

I also have my own special remedy, arrowroot, which takes its name from the arrow-shaped root of the Amaranth plant. It is sold as a fine white powder similar to cornflour and you can buy it from the home baking department of any good supermarket. It has been used since Roman times, generally as a food for invalids and babies and to alleviate the symptoms of stomach and bowel problems. It is cooling and soothing to the whole digestive system. It is my first line of defence against inflammation and I take it knowing that it soon reduces internal swelling and leads quickly to the elimination of excess water. You may have found for yourself that water retention increases the inflammation in your body. Because it is not a drug, arrowroot causes none of the nasty side effects that often accompany drugs. Arrowroot has no taste. You may know it as a thickener for soups, stews and fruit dishes, or used by itself or with cornflour to make desserts flavoured with vanilla or chocolate. I make it into a drink by mixing a heaped teaspoonful with enough cold water to make a paste, then adding hot water up to a cupful, stirring gently until it turns clear.

Other foods that will help you are described below.

Onions, shallots, spring onions and chives

These are valuable to anyone with arthritis, rheumatic pain or period pain. They ease fluid retention and promote the elimination of urea, a chemical produced by the body as part of waste elimination. A build-up of urea can make inflammatory conditions worse.

Olive oil

This has nutritional and medicinal qualities. It contains vitamins A and E and the minerals phosphorous, potassium and manganese, as well as antioxidants. The oil is useful in balancing cholesterol levels in the blood and preventing fatty deposits being laid down in the arteries and, as a consequence, may reduce heart disease, blood clots and strokes. Anyone with chronic pain needs to have good blood flow to all parts of the body and this is where olive oil plays its part. If you are changing your diet to reduce the amount of saturated fat you use in cooking or in ready-made foods then olive oil is a good substitute. When using it for stir-frying, use a little olive oil with the same amount of water. Olive oil is helpful in easing the ravages of stress and poor food absorption in the digestive system. It is often recommended as a remedy for constipation that results from the use of prescription medicines. A dessertspoonful of cold-pressed extra-virgin olive oil can be taken either by itself or drizzled on a piece of bread or toast.

Ginger

Ginger has well-known anti-inflammatory effects; it helps block the chemicals that trigger inflammation. Studies indicate that people who have migraine can be helped by taking half to one teaspoonful of ground ginger each day. I take it in this way from time to time and find that it helps in my battle against inflammation, contributing to the reduction of swelling and joint stiffness. Since digestive problems seem to accompany many of the common pain disorders it is worth using ginger as a digestive aid. It can be used either in the powdered form or as grated fresh root; the effect is the same. Besides reducing inflammation in the gut it reduces nausea and has a calming effect on the stomach and bowel, thus promoting healing. I also use root ginger liberally in cooking, sliced very thinly or grated. It is particularly good in Chinese dishes or added to marmalades or jams. My first cup of tea in the morning is lemon and ginger. It is worth trying a daily dose of ginger for yourself over a period of three months before making a judgement. Any natural remedy such as this needs time. It is not an instant fix; it is the cumulative effect that is important. There is no fear of overdosing or side effects.

Turmeric

The effects of turmeric are similar to those of ginger in that they have a calming, cooling, anti-inflammatory effect on the digestive system and bowel. There are also research indications that turmeric may be effective in preventing some forms of cancer.

Broccoli

Fortunately, broccoli is my favourite vegetable so I eat lots of it. As a bonus I find it helpful in combating fluid retention and inflammation, and consequently it is one of the weapons I use in reducing my pain. It has a high vitamin C and mineral content so it adds nutritional value to any meal.

Finally, think about setting yourself another target during the next week. It could be related to making a start on your food intake. Remember to complete your diary and look for any patterns emerging. Is your pain worse after sitting for a long period? Is your breathing more measured? Is relaxation beginning to have an impact on your pain? In view of the passage you have just read about food, why not keep a food diary so you will get some idea of your daily intake and the sort of food you are eating?

Review of Session 2

There have been many things to think about in this session as well as meeting new physical challenges. It is important that you do not feel overwhelmed so take time in the next week to go over everything at your own pace, as everyone learns differently and adapts to change in their own way. Things you may find difficult now will become easier as you practise your new skills and absorb new information. If you need two weeks before you move on to the next session then that is fine as long as you do not forget to exercise and practise relaxation daily. Slow and steady progress is what we are after. The more enjoyable experiences you can add to your life the better.

Session 3

In this session we will continue with exercise and then revise Progressive Muscle Relaxation. We will talk about understanding your pain and have a look at the question of posture. Finally, we will build upon the work started in Session 2, Activity 7.

Activity 8
Physical exercise

Start by completing the exercises outlined in Sessions 1 and 2, and when you have done those we will add some new ones.

Lower back roll

For those who feel comfortable with floor exercises, lie down with your legs together. Raise both knees towards your chest and grip them with your hands (see Figure 12). Now, gently roll over on to the right hip and then back to the centre; then to the left hip and back to the centre. Do this three times to each side.

Now, still holding your knees towards your chest, take your knees around in a circular movement.

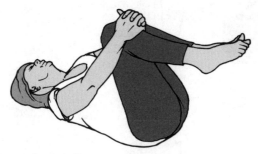

Figure 12 Lower back roll

The cat sequence

Take up the position shown in Figure 13a overleaf, with knees on the floor, slightly apart, and hands at shoulder level, with head and hands pointing forwards.

Now, breathe in and slowly raise your head and look up, while at the same time dropping the middle of the back down (see Figure 13b). Many people are very stiff in the spine so do not worry if you do not appear to drop very far. The importance of this exercise is that you make the attempt. With practice, you should find yourself loosening up. Hold this position, still looking upwards, for a count of five and then smoothly, as you let go of the breath, raise your back in an arch, at the same time bringing your head towards your knees (see Figure 13c). Repeat the sequence three times.

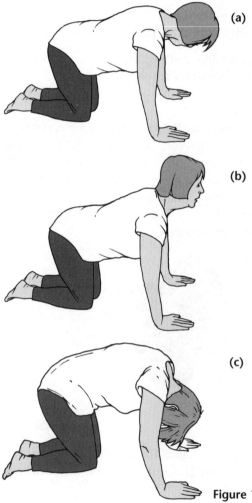

(a)

(b)

(c)

Figure 13 The cat sequence

An extension of this sequence is to move from the kneeling position (Figure 13a) and, as you breathe in, take your left knee towards your left ear with your left foot straight and flat on the floor. Now, when you feel balanced, raise both arms to the back with palms facing upwards (see Figure 14).

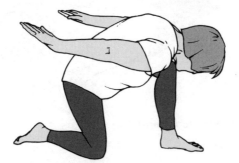

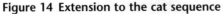

Figure 14 Extension to the cat sequence

Half press-up

Start in the relaxed position, lying flat on your stomach, with arms by your sides, palms upwards. Place your forehead on the floor and bring your arms up to shoulder level (see Figure 15). Breathe in, and slowly raise your head and look towards the ceiling. Your shoulders and chest will follow. Do not go too far to begin with. As you breathe out, slowly lower your head to the floor and place your arms back at your sides. Repeat this sequence three times – and remember, no straining.

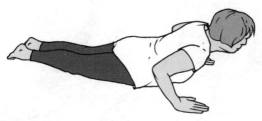

Figure 15 Half press-up

As an alternative, lie flat, with your forehead resting on the floor and your hands at shoulder level. On the in breath, lift your head a few centimetres and support your chin in your hands (see Figure

16). Hold that position for a count of five, then, on the out breath, gently remove your hands back to their original position and lower your forehead to the floor.

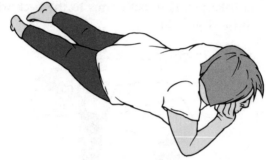

Figure 16 Half press-up (alternative)

The pose of a child

This yoga position is a good way to begin to relax. Start in a kneeling position, with knees slightly apart, and with the hands at shoulder level. Breathe in, and on the out breath sit back on your heels, lower your head to the floor and allow your arms to stretch forward (see Figure 17a). Hold this position for a few minutes and then come back up to the kneeling position. Now, sink back on your heels and bring your arms back to your sides with palms upwards (see Figure 17b).

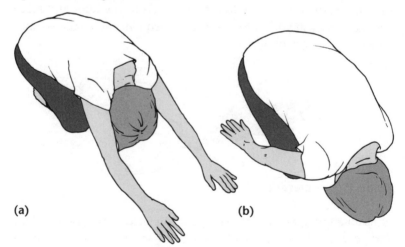

(a)   (b)

Figure 17 The pose of a child

Relaxation

When you have completed these exercises, finish off with a good floor relaxation (Figure 18). Get your blanket or duvet and cover yourself to keep warm, because you may want to stay in this position for some time.

Lie flat on your stomach, with your arms by your sides, palms upwards and with your head to one side. Breathe normally, allowing any thoughts that come flitting into your mind to pass through. Any external noises – just let them go.

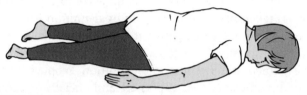

Figure 18 Relaxation

Activity 9
Progressive Muscle Relaxation

I have not forgotten that some of you cannot get down to the floor to do your exercises, so now is your chance to practise Progressive Muscle Relaxation sitting in your chair. Hopefully, you have been doing this throughout the past week. You should by now be feeling the benefit and are able to appreciate the difference between relaxed muscles and tense muscles. If you have managed the floor exercises then follow them with Progressive Muscle Relaxation as described in Session 1, Activity 4.

Topic F
Understanding your pain

For a full discussion of this topic you may like to see Chapter 1 of my book *Coping Successfully with Pain*, also published by Sheldon Press.

What is pain?

Normally, pain is a signal that the body is under attack, an alarm that calls for attention. It is part of the body's defence system and draws attention to a physical problem or injury. After treatment it usually goes away. This kind of pain is known as acute pain. Some pain arrives too late to warn us. For example, pain that may arise after a disease process is established, such as cancer pain. This type of pain might be regarded as useless pain.

Chronic pain may also be regarded as useless pain because it continues either in the absence of any illness or injury, or long after healing has taken place. Chronic pain by definition is long lasting and although not life threatening, it has the potential to be physically and emotionally destructive. This is why chronic pain should never be ignored. It is a very serious condition. People with chronic pain can become anxious, depressed and socially isolated, and may even have a breakdown in relationships as a result. It is not appropriate to treat only the anxiety or depression and expect that the pain will go away. It is a condition that needs its own special form of treatment. When chronic pain is treated appropriately, the depression and anxiety fade accordingly.

What is real pain?

All pain is real pain. All too often, people with chronic pain feel that their medical practitioners do not believe them and feel fobbed off. There is often no obvious physical cause. For many years, people with fibromyalgia were in this position until investigations led to physicians being able to describe the illness and its accompanying symptoms and problems. Recently, I heard about the case of a woman who has had chronic pain for many years. Her problem started when she strained her back at work and was advised to rest and take painkillers.

Some years later she frequently complained of back pain when lifting her children. The same advice was given and eventually the pain cleared up. A few months later she felt numbness down her thigh, and when it got worse she went to her doctor and was told she had sciatica. Again, the same treatment was given: rest and painkillers. Over a period of years she had a number of such episodes before she was told she had a disc problem. Things got so bad she had to take more and more time off work and eventually she lost her job. She had entered the chronic pain state. She has been treated for the past five years solely with painkillers and anti-depressants. The situation put a lot of strain on her marriage and recently it broke up altogether. She is now being treated for high blood pressure and diabetes.

The physiology of pain

Pain messages are conveyed by the nervous system along pathways to the brain. It is the brain that feels the pain, while the spinal cord is the main route for conveying the pain messages to and from the brain. Within the spinal cord, pain messages are passed to a fast or a slow route (called the ascending tract). The brain itself counteracts pain messages along a descending tract. Messages are transmitted to enable chemical substances to be released so that 'gates' in the spinal cord can be closed to block off ascending messages. These chemical substances are referred to as neurotransmitters and act as painkillers.

Among the neurotransmitters are the endorphins and encephalins, which have a similar effect to morphine or heroin. People differ in their capacity to produce these chemicals but exercise, relaxation, positive thinking and engaging in pleasurable activity all stimulate the production of endorphins.

Experience tells us that rubbing a painful spot reduces pain. Melzack and Wall (see Further reading) propounded a theory to account for this, suggesting that the rubbing produces a sensation that is conveyed faster than the pain message, telling the brain to give the signal to 'close the gate' to any pain message being conveyed towards it. Very often when I am experiencing pain walking I find the nearest tree and rub my spine up and down the trunk. It is not very good for my clothes but it is very effective in closing the gate on my pain.

Coping with pain

Medication that is effective in acute pain is not really appropriate for the treatment of chronic pain, as its long-term use is damaging to the digestive system, liver and kidneys. I know of many instances when stronger drugs are used or dosages are increased when people with chronic pain fail to respond to the medication. The result can be toxicity, physical damage, an increase in pain and even psychological damage. The mechanism that triggers the brain to produce endorphins is suppressed and the 'gates' remain open, allowing the pain messages to get through.

Our capacity to cope with pain is reduced by prolonged inactivity, drug dependency, toxicity, negative feelings or stressful experiences. Anticipation of pain, along with imagination and painful memories, can help trigger physiological changes that make pain real, and even intensify it.

It helps to think of each pain episode as an isolated event that has nothing to do with the past and nothing to do with anything that is likely to happen in the future. The memory of past pain and the anticipation of future pain can make an episode feel so much worse. If you break your arm you can have a lot of pain, but you experience no lasting psychological or emotional distress. You know the pain will go away as soon as the arm is mended. You have to play a psychological trick on yourself and learn to treat your chronic pain in the same way. Learn to accept that your pain will come – and your pain will go. A minority of people have pain all of the time and learn how to ignore it.

Good relaxation can help reduce sensitivity and the number and length of pain episodes you experience. This is why so much emphasis is placed in this book on various ways of achieving deep relaxation.

Pain and suffering

Pain and the feelings being experienced may not be obvious to an onlooker because many people show no external signs of their problem. Even professionals may find it difficult to accept that a person who appears to be a healthy individual has a serious pain problem, and so we may find alternative ways of presenting our pain.

We all give off signals verbally, facially and through body language about the way we feel. You can tell when someone is angry by how they tighten their mouth and get a bit red in the face. Then again, a young woman in love positively glows and chatters to anyone who will listen about the wonderful man who has entered her life.

Learn to distinguish between your pain and your suffering. Without displays of suffering, your pain can go unnoticed. Suffering is the outward and visible sign that you are in a state of dis-ease. For example, a grieving person shows signs of suffering possibly by weeping, becoming easily upset and turning away from friendly gestures. Pain, on the other hand, is an illness that has physical, emotional, psychological and social implications and is therefore a very serious condition; without displays of suffering it is possible that some or all of these implications will remain untreated. You cannot see it, you cannot bandage it, you may have had a number of operations and be on a regime of tablets, but still the pain persists.

This passage is as difficult for me to write as it may be for you to accept, because in many ways it is a description that could apply to any of us who have chronic pain.

Suffering is signalled by behaviour. Gasps, sighs, holding parts of the body, awkward walking, outbursts of impatience, tearfulness, being grouchy or silent for long periods, going to bed and withdrawing from company are all common signals. Displays of suffering disturb family, social and work relationships. When I had my hypnotherapy practice I used to watch some clients leave their car quite cheerfully and walk quite normally. By the time they reached my front door they had adopted a hangdog expression and developed an awkward gait. Perhaps they thought that unless I saw them suffering I would not believe they were in pain.

Suffering is not necessarily proportional to the amount of pain being experienced. Suffering seems to be magnified by strong negative feelings. These may result from losing a job, money worries, losing mobility and the many other losses that result from having chronic pain. The situation is made much more difficult if medical advisers can give no indication when your pain will be over or they appear to have washed their hands of you.

Over the years I have learned that displays of suffering are unhelpful, as they take a lot of energy and keep your mind firmly focused on the pain. These displays can be very destructive to family relationships. I know of a number of marriage breakups in which the partner has found the burden of constantly adapting to the behaviour and moods of the 'pain sufferer' just too much. It is so easy to feel, as a partner, that you are in some way responsible for the suffering. The dynamics of the relationship can change: no companionship, possibly no normal family life, financial burdens, difficulty with care of children and no time to devote to anyone else, neglect of house and garden or no family holidays. The family becomes virtually a one-parent household with an adult dependant. It needs a lot of strength to cope in these circumstances. Should there be a family breakup then the person with pain really does have problems.

Having your pain recognized

It is very important that chronic pain is recognized and treated early. Treatment needs to focus on every aspect of a person's life and be concentrated on maintaining mobility, functioning socially outside and inside the family, dealing with anxiety, depression and sleeplessness where it applies and, of course, providing a repertoire of resources to cope with the pain. This is a lot to ask of the NHS so it is important that we take responsibility for our own well-being.

The fact that pain can be invisible to others can often place the person with pain in a quandary. How can you communicate to others that you have pain and need some consideration, without displays of suffering? It is important for you to become aware of how you communicate the fact that you have pain to other people. It is also important that you work towards reducing conscious and unconscious signals of suffering. By ridding yourself of these you can go a long way to reducing the amount of pain you experience. This is difficult psychological territory, as mind and body are so closely interlinked. If you have ever done any acting you will know how, by adopting the role of an old, sick person, your own posture and the way you feel can change dramatically and it can take some time to recover from the part. By acting as though you have no pain you can bring about changes in the way you think, the way you feel and the way you behave. It is well worth making the changes, in spite of the fact that you may feel your audience still needs to maintain its belief that you have an illness.

Do your utmost to be cheerful, upright in posture and well-groomed, so that even close relatives can be fooled. In working hard to fool others you can in fact fool yourself. I have always devoted time in the group situation to help people learn acting skills to enable them to show a positive face to the world. Just for a moment imagine you are sitting on a train going to London to collect your lottery winnings. How are you sitting? What expression is on your face? Now bring to mind a different scenario, one that happened to me recently; you reach into your pocket to pay for a meal and find that your wallet has gone and with it your cash and credit cards. What is the expression on your face now?

In spite of all that I have said, the reality is that pain is invisible, and although you may look fit you may also be rather fragile, have poor balance, low energy and be vulnerable when out on the street. It would be inappropriate to carry a bell, as did the lepers of old, or have 'chronic pain sufferer' stamped on your forehead, so it seems perfectly legitimate to have a way of signalling to others to take care. This signal may take the form of a stick, elbow crutches or some other support.

Do not be a sufferer

As part of your homework for the next week, make a note of all the different ways you display your suffering to other people. What do you do to attract attention to yourself in order to get help or sympathy, or perhaps change the focus of conversation. Make a note of how often your conversation is dominated by the talk of pain – your pain particularly. Talking constantly of your pain and suffering can be very wearing for your audience and you may find that quite soon people prefer to seek out more entertaining company.

As an exercise with a group I once worked with, I suggested that over the lunch break the topic of pain should be excluded from all conversation. Everyone was back from lunch early! As the weeks went on everyone worked hard to find alternative discussion points for the lunch breaks, and the general feedback was that all the members of the group had come to know each other much better and wanted to know about where they lived, their family and their interests, and genuine friendships developed. They were no longer 'pain sufferers' but personalities. This change in the relationships between the members was obvious during group discussion and everyone was much more positive and enthusiastic about how they could make the changes that would make such a difference to their lives. They were even able to joke about some of the behaviour they had unconsciously adopted to remind others of their pain. One member had demonstrated to all that her pain must be worse than anyone else's by remaining steadfastly anchored to her wheel-chair and she only needed to raise her eyes to one of the helpers, who was by her side in a moment. All of us thought that she was not capable of standing or walking unsupported, but as the group changed its focus and we became more comfortable with each other, the wheelchair lost its importance and she was soon sitting in an ordinary chair within the group and taking a full part in all the activities.

Just see what happens when you exclude pain from your conversation. Think about what you will say when someone says to you: 'How is your back today?' or 'Have you been to the hospital lately?' When people address you in this way it is demonstrating how they see you. It is also a lazy way for them to open a conversation. It is as automatic a conversation opener as the hairdresser asking if you have been on holiday. When someone asks how you are, instead of reciting a list of aches and pains, just say, 'Fine, thanks' and be ready with a question for them. Refuse to be drawn into any conversation which involves you doing most of the talking – about your pain. If you are in a group with other people who have pain, make it clear that pain is not on your agenda for conversation. If you need help, then ask for it directly. Do not expect people who have no training to know exactly how you are feeling at any moment. As you make these changes, note how other people's behaviour changes towards you.

Activity 10
Exercise leading into relaxation

This activity builds on Session 2, Activity 7, so begin by following the instructions for that activity, then continue as follows:

1 I want you to repeat the arm-raising exercise but now breathe in to a count of four and out to a count of eight. You will have to slow down your out breath and keep it in time with the lowering of your arms. Aim to have them half way by the count of four. At

first you may feel that you are running out of breath but as you synchronize the movement to the breath it will become easier. With practice, you will be able to manage an in breath of six and an out breath of 18. But for the moment we will concentrate on four in and eight out. When you can manage this please repeat the exercise twice more.

2 Now we are going to try a count of six in and eight out, so, breathing in to a count of six, raise the arms over the head and clasp them together. Hold the clasp and the breath for a count of four then lower the arms to the sides to a count of eight. Repeat twice more. Now, draw the shoulders up to the ears, hold for a count of five, then drop them down quickly. Shake out hands, arms, feet and legs until all tension is gone.

3 Place the hands, with palms in the prayer position, in the middle of the chest. Breathe in to a count of four, at the same time pressing the palms together and putting tension on the upper arms and shoulders. Hold for a count of five then breathe out, relaxing the hands. Repeat twice more.

4 Again, place the hands with palms together in the prayer position. Now, to a count of four breathe in and raise the hands together until the arms are straight above the head. Hold for a count of five, then breathe out, lowering the arms and hands to the starting position. Shake out the hands and arms before repeating twice more.

5 As an alternative to step 5, place the palms together in front of you close to the chest. Keeping the palms together, but this time with fingers pointing forwards, and breathing in to a count of four, push the arms forward from the body until they are fully extended. Hold for a count of five and then, as you breathe out to a count of four, return your hands and arms to their original position in front of the chest. Repeat twice more.

6 Stand with palms together as in step 6. Now, keeping the palms together extend the arms out in front of you, at the same time breathe in to a count of four. Keeping the arms extended and breathing out, press the left palm against the right one and push the arms over to the right about 15 cm (6 inches) and stop. Breathe in and return the hands to the centre and apply pressure with the opposite hand. As this is a strong exercise there are no repeats.

7 Stand upright with the feet about 23 cm (9 inches) apart. Look straight ahead to a point on the wall in front of you. Keep your arms relaxed at the sides and, as you breathe in to a count of four, slowly move the head to the left, halfway between the front and the side. Hold for a count of five, then on the out breath, to a count of four, return the head to the front. Repeat the movement to the left and, still breathing in to a count of four, move the head slightly further around towards the side. Hold the breath for a count of five and as you breathe out to a count of four move the head to the front. Repeat this movement to the same side and as you breathe in, move the head as far as possible to the left, hold the position for a count of five and on the out breath slowly take the head around to face the front.

8 Repeat step 7 to the right side.

Remain in the balanced position enjoying the feeling of warmth resulting from the release of tension from the neck and shoulder muscles. To finish, bring your shoulders up towards your ears, hold the position for a count of five then quickly drop your shoulders, releasing the tension. In Session 4 this activity will be extended to complete Exercise leading into relaxation.

At this point you may wish to lie down on the floor and cover yourself with a blanket and just enjoy the feeling of relaxation as you practice your diaphragmatic breathing.

Topic G
Posture and movement

Bad posture plays an important part in contributing to pain. Conversely, good posture can do much to alleviate pain and prevent tensions on the body, which are at the root of wear and tear. Unfortunately, people with painful conditions may be reaping the results of many years of standing and sitting incorrectly.

Bad posture may result from injury problems, ill-fitting shoes, sitting or standing in one position for too long, adjusting your body position to ease pain, stooping to guard against pain, sitting with legs crossed or one leg extended or held stiffly, or reclining for long periods on a soft couch.

Bad posture is the main reason for neck pain. We often sit with our head tilted backwards or bent forwards. I heard a comment the other day from a chiropractor, who said that tilting the head forwards by just 8 cm (3 inches) can increase the weight of the head threefold (the average human head weighs about 5 kg or 11 lbs.) So just think how much strain this imposes on your neck and spine and how much energy is used just to hold it up. Sleeping with a pile of pillows can also push the head forwards, leading to head and neck pain. Try making sure that your neck is fully supported when you are asleep. Use a rolled-up towel to fill in the gap between the shoulder and neck, or use one of the posture pillows on the market. The head and neck exercises in Activity 10 will be very helpful to anyone who has head and neck pain.

Bad posture increases tension

Bad posture places undue tension on individual muscles or groups of muscles, which work to compensate for the strain that is being placed on the body. Any muscle held under tension for a long time can produce pain and discomfort. The release of tension often causes the muscle to go into spasm.

Adopting good habits can bring about dramatic improvement in the frequency and severity of pain. However, before you can make permanent and effective changes you need to become aware of your existing habits. How do you sit? What sort of chair do you sit on? What position do you adopt to watch TV or to read? Are you in the sort of job where you have to sit or stand for long periods or adopt a sideways or tilting position to manipulate tools? Do you spend long periods washing-up at a sink that is too low? Are you working in a job which demands that your hands and arms need to be above your head for long periods? If you are in such a job then it is important that, if these positions cannot be avoided, that you exercise at least once an hour to relieve the unnatural tensions that build up.

Bad posture eats up your energy and this is more marked in people with pain. In the previous pages I talked about pain behaviour and displays of suffering, many of which involve adopting difficult body positions, bending, tilting and limping. These changes in posture are extremely energy-sapping. Most of the exercises in this book will help to make a big difference to your posture and do much to preserve your energy.

Balanced sitting position

You can begin to make a big difference by sitting in a balanced position. You will have noticed that the relaxation instructions always begin by asking you to adopt a 'balanced sitting position'. This is illustrated in Figure 19. As you sit down, make sure that your bottom leads the way to the back of the seat. Avoid flopping straight down and leaving a gap between the bottom of your spine and the back of the seat. Ensure that you sit with your knees bent, your thighs parallel with the floor and your feet flat. Do not tilt your head backwards or forwards but keep your chin parallel with the floor. Whenever I work with a group I make a point of asking people to sit without their legs crossed and ask the members to point out at any time when others are sitting in this way, including myself.

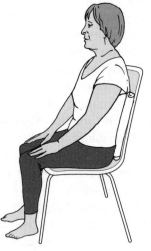

Figure 19 Balanced sitting position

Standing up from a sitting position

Getting out of a chair is equally important. If you are working with a group, ask each one in turn to get up and walk across the room. Most people start moving forward before they have completed the rise from the seat. You will notice a number of them will hold their back or side, grimace, or continue to walk in an ungainly or stooped way. It is useful to spend time learning to rise in a balanced and graceful way. When preparing to get up, move one foot slightly in front of the other. Place your hands on the seat at each side of your body, lean forwards and, taking your weight on your hands and then your feet, raise your body to an upright position. Some people find it easier to place their hands on their knees rather than on the seat. Pause in the standing position, breathe into the diaphragm as you pause, look straight ahead and fix your eyes on a point at the other side of the room and only then, walk forwards with the head erect. This may involve a number of repetitions to get the movement right, but it is worth it.

If you are leading a group, ask the members in turn to walk across the room and invite the other members to observe each walk closely, looking out for raised tense shoulders. This may be a sign that someone is accustomed to carrying a shoulder bag or perhaps it is from many hours leaning over a desk or a computer. Notice whether feet tilt over on shoes that have worn down. After a few months, shoes get distorted as a result of bad walking practice and no longer give adequate support. Suggest having new shoes more often and in particular having the feet measured before buying shoes. Some people go on buying the same type of shoe irrespective of changes in the body. Note whether people are wearing extremely flat shoes. Shoes that are too flat are not helpful to the balance of people with spinal problems, arthritis and sciatica. They can also put undue strain on the lower back and can aggravate back pain. Just as bad are low-cut high-heeled shoes which force the wearer to teeter along holding themselves in a tense position to keep them on. This tension is felt throughout the body. Suggest shoes that are designed specifically to absorb shock.

Anyone who has an unbalanced walk will be helped considerably by being encouraged to pause before they start walking, adopt diaphragmatic breathing and look straight ahead before setting off. With practice, it is possible that everyone will notice considerable improvement. It is worth repeating this activity on a number of occasions throughout the course to see if bad habits are returning and, of course, to recognize the improvements. This session is well worth recording on video so that members can see for themselves how they sit and how they walk. An individual can learn very rapidly to make improvements as a result of seeing video playback. It may take a couple of hours to complete this activity.

If you are working alone it can be helpful to walk towards a full-length mirror. Even just standing in front of the mirror can show up a lifted shoulder, a tilt to one side or a chin too high. It helps to get a partner or friend to work with you on this activity and ask them to be honest and point out any signs they notice that your bodyline is out of balance.

Review of Session 3

During the session you have been asked to work very hard, extending your physical capabilities so that you can become more flexible and have more stamina and energy. As a bonus you will be gaining confidence and others will begin to notice improvements in your appearance. The session has given you an opportunity to develop your relaxation skills and you have learned how exercise itself will naturally lead into a release of tension and consequently a decrease in pain. You have been asked to consider how you present yourself to other people by becoming aware of your own body language and the signals you display. You may have found this hard to take. I know I certainly did when asked to undertake this exercise but, having done it, had to admit that it marked a big step forward in my progress. So, in the few days before moving on to Session 4, continue to practise and enjoy your daily physical exercises. Develop your relaxation skills once or twice a day, especially at bedtime and after you have been shopping or doing housework or have been involved in a tense situation at work. Continue to pay attention to your posture and movement and, finally, record your progress in your diary.

Session 4

In this session we will continue to focus attention on exercise and relaxation, building on the work in the previous three sessions. We will look at ways of thinking and behaving more positively and changing the way we relate to others. You will be asked to provide your own ideas because you know best what pushes your buttons.

Activity 11
Physical exercise

Go through all of the exercises outlined in the first three sessions. By this time you should be fit and confident enough to repeat each exercise at least twice as many times as you did in the first session without strain or undue fatigue. Do not rush them, take your time, and stop if you feel any discomfort. If you have been spending a week between each session and exercising daily, your level of fitness must have improved and you are now probably ready to take on some physical challenges such as walking, swimming or pool exercises, cycling (I use an exercise bike on wet or cold days) or think about joining a yoga or t'ai chi class in your area.

Yoga

Yoga has been used for many years for healing and there is evidence that it can help relieve symptoms over a wide range of disorders. A course of yoga helps bring about physical and mental improvements through learning a series of physical postures and controlled breathing exercises. People with poor mobility as a result of pain can be helped to regain physical fitness through a series of gentle exercises which involve no strain. Many people find it helpful as a form of meditation, helping them to achieve relaxation and feelings of well-being. A study in 2004 in New Jersey showed that a six-week course of yoga was successful in treating 22 patients with low back pain. It has also been shown to relieve fatigue in people with multiple sclerosis. Information about finding a yoga teacher near to you will be found in the Useful addresses section at the end of the book. People with back or eye problems, hypertension, clotting disorders, thrombosis or osteoporosis should avoid inverted postures such as head or shoulder stands. It is important that you make your teacher fully aware of your medical condition before you start any course of physical exercise.

T'ai chi

T'ai chi is a form of qigong, which means 'working with energy'. It is an ancient system of exercise combining movement, breath and meditation. The t'ai chi exercises are done very slowly and smoothly. They are particularly good for older people or people with mobility problems who might have difficulties with balance. From experience I know they are very relaxing and have been described as a form of moving meditation. T'ai chi would make a very good progression if you want to continue beyond this book.

Activity 12
Relaxation and visualization

Emotions and thoughts can have a profound effect on physical and mental health. Feeling relaxed and in control can help improve our well-being and promote healing. A number of studies have shown that visualization, which enables people to experience beneficial emotional states, can bring about improvements for people with anxiety, pain and even physical problems such as asthma and arthritis. For this reason, I need to show you how you can begin to practise this form of therapy for yourself.

From now on, during this course, relaxation training will take place with you sitting in a balanced position in a chair. Remember to tuck your bottom well into the back of the chair, place your feet together flat on the floor (no crossed legs) and let your hands rest gently on your thighs. Make sure your head and neck are well supported. If you have a tendency to slump to one side, support yourself with a cushion or pillow. During relaxation there is a tendency to cool down so cover yourself and keep warm.

By now it may be possible for you to be able to develop the state of relaxation for yourself, without any instructions. Remember to slow down your breathing and focus your breath into your diaphragm, making your out breath longer than your in breath. As your breathing becomes slower and deeper, just allow any stray thoughts that come into your mind to pass through – don't dwell on them . . . . For the next few minutes I am going to show you a way to harness those resources deep within yourself that can help with your healing . . . . . so continue to breathe slowly and deeply and allow your relaxation to develop . . . .

I believe someone once said that the most important pictures we can see are the ones behind our eyes. Most of us are able to visualize, to see pictures in our mind's eye. Unfortunately, some people have pictures pop into their minds at random and they are not necessarily pictures they want to be reminded of. In the last session the relaxation exercise involved recalling good memories because these can have a profound effect on the way we feel and the way we behave. As a hypnotherapist I encourage clients to develop visualization as it is a powerful tool in healing so I want to help you to develop this skill for yourself. Visualization is most effective during deep relaxation, when the body and mind are completely at rest. That state, between waking and sleeping – drifting – is a state we've all experienced.

We have spent a lot of time working on Progressive Muscle Relaxation, which involved some physical action followed by relaxation. This time I would like you to achieve the state of relaxation without any physical effort whatever. Just focus on your breathing into the diaphragm, making the out breath longer than the in breath. Continue this way for a few minutes, making your breathing slower . . . . . . and deeper . . . .

Focus your attention on the top of your head . . . . Do you feel any tension there? If you do, just think about . . . . . . letting it go (you don't have to do anything physically). Now, focus on your forehead . . . . . It is surprising how often we frown or build up tension in this area when we are reading, or driving or listening to what people are saying and this tension can spread throughout the body . . . . . So focus on this area and just let the brow smooth out . . . . . . release the tension, and likewise the eyes – let any tension move away from there. Now, think about the face and the jaw . . . . Are your teeth clenched . . .? Let them part a little and drop your tongue to the bottom of your mouth . . . . Let all the tension move away from this area . . . . and the neck . . . . . . and

shoulders . . . . . . release the tension . . . and the arms . . . . . . the wrists
. . . . . . the hands and fingers . . . . let all the tension drain away . . . .
By now it may be possible to experience the warmth of increased blood
flow through your arms, to the hands, and this is good . . . . Enjoy the
feeling for a few moments . . . . . Now, focus on the spine and the long
muscles on either side of the spine; these can become very tense . . . . .
So let the tension go from here . . . . . . and the muscles of the chest
. . . . . . the stomach . . . . . . and the pelvis . . . Let the tension go . . . . .
Now your buttocks and thighs . . . . . . all around your knees . . . . . .
your calves . . . . . . ankles, feet and toes . . . . . . let all the remaining
tension drain away through the ends of your toes . . . . . Experience for
some moments the warmth of relaxation spread throughout your body
. . . .

This is the time to bring to mind an image of yourself when you felt
at your best, your most proud, your most confident . . . . . . Make that
picture as bright and as big as you possibly can and remember too how
you felt at that time . . . . . . How were you dressed . . .? What sort of
day was it . . .? Who were you with . . .? Take your time and enjoy every
aspect of that experience . . . . . . hearing the sounds associated with it
. . . . . . Make your picture as vivid as possible . . . . . . and enjoy once
more the feeling of well-being that it brought . . . . . Spend some time
relaxing in this way because this is the most important thing you can be
doing right now . . . .

When you are ready, and only when you are ready . . . . . slowly become
aware of sounds around you and know that you can benefit from this
good experience and enjoy an increased sense of well-being any time
you wish to return to this state of relaxation . . . . . or even sit quietly
in that special place you have set aside for yourself . . . . . . return to a
state of full awareness feeling so much more confident, invigorated and
comfortable in your body . . . . When you are ready just open your eyes
and begin to move your hands . . . . . . your arms . . . . . . and your feet
. . . . . . and now slowly stand up and move around.

Topic H
Beginning to think and behave in a positive way

This section is continued from Session 2, Topic D.

Pain can destroy social relationships. Many problems that people
with pain experience result from isolation. Because of your illness

you may have had to withdraw from work; even if you are at work you may spend time wrapped in your own thoughts. There, but not there. You shut people out. You are unwilling to take part in social activities. You no longer go to the pub or your favourite club. You stop inviting people to your home and, without realizing it, you become totally absorbed in your pain. The more isolated you become the more your thinking becomes negative and you may easily be provoked to anger.

Anger often accompanies the pain state. It may not be expressed directly but may be the emotion that underlies a growing state of apparent depression. Anyone with pain has a right to feel angry because many things that you have cherished have been lost as a result of experiencing chronic pain. You can quite easily list those things: a promotion, a job, income, status in the outside world and possibly within the family. Relationships might have suffered or even broken down completely. You may have lost the pleasure you get from being involved in simple games, pastimes and outings with your children. If you bury the anger and do not acknowledge it, it can lead to a deep depression and it can also colour virtually every relationship.

Make a list of all the things you have lost as a result of your pain and, alongside each of the items you mention, make a few comments on how you feel. You may find this difficult but it is well worth the effort because this can be the start of the healing process.

When you are fit and pain-free you are probably not easily upset by the thoughtless or even rude things people say or do. Illness of any kind makes people sensitive or touchy. You will have noticed that so far in the course we have spent time cultivating positive feelings. Being able to relax completely is a very positive activity, which has the effect of resting the mind and the body. It is during these periods of relaxation that you can begin to think of how you might change the way you relate and respond to others. The whole process starts very simply but it does involve thinking in advance about how you deal with certain situations or comments.

Here is an exercise that many have found helpful:

Take a few moments and establish your breathing into your diaphragm. Slowly breathe in . . . . slowly breathe out . . . for about ten full breaths

. . . . . . if you have not done so already . . . . allow your eyes to close . . . . breathe more deeply and slowly . . . Now is the time to call upon one of your strongest allies to help you sort out your problem . . . . . . you know what that problem is . . . . you know that you are having difficulty coping in a certain situation . . . . or in the way you get on with other people or perhaps one person in particular . . . . . Continue breathing in this relaxing . . . . peaceful . . . . calming way . . . and remember . . . . you have an unconscious mind that ever since you were born . . . has looked after you in many ways without you even being aware of it . . . . Your eyes can blink . . . to protect you from dust . . . If you are a cyclist you ride without even thinking how to balance. You can no doubt think of many ways your unconscious mind helps you get through the day without you being aware . . . . . . You are sitting now, you are breathing and your temperature has adjusted to suit the conditions in the room . . . . so trust your unconscious mind to help you find a solution to your problem . . .

Continue to think about the help you need and ask the part of your mind that can help you . . . . . to find a solution . . . . Taking your time . . . . . feeling very comfortable . . . you may experience some feeling within you that your unconscious mind has taken on this task . . . . you may visualize the solution or it may be that within the next few days, without even thinking about it, you meet a situation or person you have been worrying about . . . . and behave quite differently . . . . feeling comfortable and relaxed . . . . about it . . . . . Just continue to enjoy this comfortable state for a few minutes . . . . . . while your unconscious mind works away on your behalf . . . . In your own good time . . . become aware of your surroundings and feeling refreshed and full of energy . . . open your eyes.

Activity 13
Exercise leading into relaxation

If you can manage it, repeat Activity 7 in Session 2 and then Activity 10 in Session 3 and continue with the new exercise below. By combining the three exercises you will have given yourself a complete workout without too much effort. However, you can benefit by doing this new exercise on its own. This concentrates on unwinding the top half of the body while putting tension on the legs and hamstrings. *Anyone who feels dizzy or otherwise uncomfortable during this exercise should stop immediately and sit down.*

1 Standing in the balanced position, with knees locked and arms hanging by the sides, breathe in, and now very slowly as you breathe out lower the head, shoulders and each vertebra, one at a time, lowering the head, the shoulders, the upper spine until the top half of the body is hanging over like a rag doll, with arms flopping loosely. There should be no tension in the body except for the legs. The more slowly you do this exercise the more effective it will be.

2 Breathe normally, and when you feel you have been in the hanging position for long enough (the more you practise this movement the more comfortable you will feel and you will be able to stay hanging for longer) very slowly unwind your body from the lowest part of your spine and gradually carry on unwinding until you get to the stage where your chin is resting on your chest. Last of all, slowly raise your head until your chin is parallel with the floor.

3 Then, shrug your shoulders up to your ears and release several times.

4 Finally, breathe into the diaphragm and as you breathe out produce a sound from deep within yourself. It can be a laugh, a shout or a musical note. Just let's hear from you. Producing sound in this way is a very effective release of inner tension. It is a very enjoyable exercise, especially in a group situation. It works very well if the leader demonstrates the sound first. It might be an aaaaaahhhhh! or a mmmmmmm! or even an oooooooooo! It is even more effective if the sound is repeated over and over without a break. As you run out of breath, take a breath in and start again. As people will run out of breath at different times you get a rolling sound which vibrates around you. Besides relieving tension from deep within ourselves, laughter, singing and shouting have a profound effect on the production of endorphins, nature's pain relievers and mood elevators.

5 Complete this exercise by taking time to sit in a chair and relax completely.

By now you should know how to enter a state of complete relaxation. Remember, it begins with your breathing. You may allow positive images to come into your mind. Perhaps you might take the opportunity to visualize taking part in an enjoyable activity with other people. This can be a memory of some event from the past or you might like to project yourself into the future and see a fitter, more active you looking your very best with a new hairstyle (unless you are bald-headed like me), wearing your smartest clothes and oozing confidence as you set out to enjoy yourself.

This session has taken you much further with physical challenges and extended your relaxation skills, giving you an insight as to how your mind can influence the way you feel and the way you behave. You have been challenged to come out of your isolation and let your voice be heard. It will be interesting to see what you have achieved by the time you move on to Session 5.

Session 5

Session 5 involves physical exercise and continues with relaxation and visualization. The topics for this session will include looking at confidence and self-esteem and then we will move on to examining pain in relation to depression, anxiety and sleep.

Activity 14
Physical exercise

In this session I would like you to continue with all of the physical exercises described in the previous sessions. If you have been practising daily then you should be managing them all quite comfortably and have increased the repetitions considerably. You will note that the exercises can now take up quite a lot of time, so pace yourself and rest frequently. You are not involved in a competition. The amount of time you take is not important. What does matter is that you complete the exercises and enjoy the physical well-being that results.

Activity 15
Relaxation

Prepare yourself for relaxation by sitting comfortably in a chair, making sure you are well supported and covered by a duvet or blanket.

> For the next half hour you are not going anywhere, you are not going to do anything, you don't even need to think . . . All you have to do is relax completely . . . You know by now how to do this, so begin to breathe as you have been taught, into the diaphragm, allowing the out breath to be longer than the in breath . . . . slow down your breathing and gradually . . . . make it deeper . . . Now, mentally scan your body for any signs of tension, focusing on the head . . . . . . around the eyes . . . . the cheeks . . . . . . the jaw . . . . neck and shoulders . . . . the arms . . . . hands . . . . . . chest . . . . back . . . . pelvic area . . . . buttocks and thighs . . . .

73

legs . . . . . . ankles and feet . . . . . . Just feel the warmth of relaxation spreading right through your body as the tension drains away . . . . For the next few minutes I want to talk to you about a man I know . . . For many years he felt uneasy in himself. He did not know why, but things just did not go right for him and he felt bad . . . . . Most days he spent worrying about this . . . . . . then one day he noticed that because he had spent so long worrying he had neglected to look after his house . . . . he looked around and saw the clutter . . . . . . the dust . . . . . . the cobwebs . . . . . . and he thought it might be a good idea . . . . to have a spring clean.

He decided to start in the attic . . . . and that really was cluttered . . . He had intended to move much of the clutter from downstairs into the attic but there was no room . . . . it was so full of clutter he was unable to see anything of value and so he spent the day clearing out the attic . . . . . . making space and letting light in . . . . He found . . . . . . a load of rubbish . . . . broken things . . . . useless things . . . . old packaging . . . . things of little value that take a lot of space . . . . . . As he cleared out the clutter he began to feel better . . . . and he began to discover some very useful things that he had long forgotten about . . . . things that could be of use to him now and in the future . . . . tools . . . . . . valuable tools . . . . that could help him put his house in order . . . . . . He was pleased with his day's work . . . . and he set about next day . . . . with a lot of energy . . . . . and in no time at all . . . . had cleared the clutter from downstairs . . . . throwing out what he knew he would never need again . . . . and he was able to see precisely what things he would need to hold on to . . . . . . When he had finished he looked at his handiwork . . . . . . he looked at his home . . . . now smart and clean . . . . . . and he began to feel . . . . so much better . . . . much less confused . . . . knowing he could put his hand on things he might need at any time.

Just continue to enjoy the warmth . . . . . . the good feelings . . . . of relaxation . . . . knowing that you can return . . . . . . at any time . . . . to this pleasant state . . . . . . this comfortable state . . . . . . drifting . . . . . . between waking . . . . . . and sleeping . . . . . . Now pause for two minutes to allow relaxation to continue . . . When you are ready . . . . . . and only when you are ready . . . . . . slowly become aware of where you are . . . . . . begin to move your hands . . . . . . your feet . . . . . . and carrying your good feelings with you . . . . . . open your eyes . . . . . fully awake . . . . . full of energy and confidence.

Topic I
Confidence and self-esteem

It may be that your pain has shattered your confidence and lowered your self-esteem to such an extent that you have, as we explored in the previous session, found it increasingly difficult to communicate with others, make decisions or assert yourself in a way that is acceptable to those around you. We have already looked at the way in which your attitudes and emotional responses may hinder your attempts to get on with others or make positive changes. Many of your attitudes and emotional responses result not directly from your pain; for many years you may have harboured some inner discomfort that adds to your tension and, consequently, your pain. It *can* happen and you may not be in full control of your life.

I want to try to help you to identify the source of this discomfort – other people, hangovers from the past, your previous learning, or attitudes and beliefs passed on to you when you were a child. Any of these can be a major source of stress and hinder your attempts at managing your pain. I have prepared a list of statements that may or may not apply to you. Study them, think about them and see how many of the statements apply to you. Some will apply to all of us but if you find yourself agreeing with most of them then it is time to make changes, for your own benefit. It is important to acknowledge which aspects of living are contributing to your distress and feeding your pain. The following statements may be helpful in sorting out what is limiting your ability to help yourself:

- I believe there may be something basically wrong with me that is making me unhappy.
- I feel guilty when I am having my own way, even over something trivial.
- I do not like to 'rock the boat' even when something does not seem right.
- I feel guilty when I shirk a domestic duty – neglect to clean the house, leave the washing-up overnight, do not have meals ready on time.
- I feel uneasy if my partner does not have a meal ready for me when I come home.

- I think I should be able to cope with any situation and that it is a sign of failure to ask for help.
- I believe that in politics, business and science, men are naturally smarter.
- An inner voice tells me that it is the job of a 'good woman' always to look after her man.
- I believe I am not allowed to show anger. I feel angry about my situation but feel I cannot talk about it.
- I feel guilty about spending money on myself unless I have some else's approval.
- I still seek the approval, not just the advice, of my parents for major decisions in my life.
- I find it hard to accept compliments. I often think they are insincere.
- I would do almost anything to avoid an argument or confrontation.
- When I engage in conversation I emphasize key words in my sentences to get my point across.
- When talking I end my sentences very rapidly so that I can move on to other topics.
- I get impatient when other people talk and find myself finishing their sentences for them – or I interrupt before they finish.
- I rush meals so that I can get on with other things.
- I find most people work too slowly for my liking.
- I get irritated when driving if the car in front is going too slowly.
- I get irritated when I have to queue for anything, for example at a supermarket checkout.
- My mother or father come to mind when I 'disobey' a rule that they taught me as a child, and I expect to be punished.
- I believe that all rules need to be followed because they are made by people whose judgement is better than mine.
- I accept invitations to do things with friends or family even when I would rather not, and resent them for aggravating my pain.
- I attend meetings, weddings, funerals and social functions because others expect me to and not because I want to.
- If I am enjoying myself I expect discomfort to follow automatically, so I turn down opportunities to go out.

- I am afraid to try anything new in case I fail and make a fool of myself.
- I resist new experiences and have not done anything different for more than a month (if you have been sticking with this course for the last few weeks then that is a good sign).
- I feel guilty and uneasy if I am away from home for too long and I feel upset when something disrupts my daily routine.
- I feel that others do not believe that my pain is as bad as I make out and I find myself talking about it frequently to convince them.
- I tackle DIY jobs because I think it is expected of me, even although I know I am not up to it.
- I truly feel that sacrificing myself for others makes me a better person, even if it means ignoring my own needs.
- I jump up immediately to answer the doorbell or telephone. I drop everything to respond to an immediate demand.
- I am staying in a bad relationship because I would not know where to turn if I were alone.
- I am afraid to make positive steps to improve my condition because I feel I will lose out in other ways.

Once, when discussing the questionnaire, one of the group members owned up to the fact that all through her married life she had had to make soup for her husband, who demanded it at 9 o'clock every evening. It was his belief that he could not go a day without his soup so, for 40 years, she had followed this pattern. The soup habit had been established by his mother who had served soup to the family every night for supper. The questionnaire had helped her to realize just how much she resented doing this. The group spent a long time discussing how she could change the pattern and she went off home with the suggestion that she should tell her husband directly that she was no longer going to make soup on a daily basis. This she did and was surprised when he replied: 'Oh, I look forward to a change. I didn't like to ask you why it was always soup for supper.' He had long since forgotten what he had told her all those years ago.

Another woman in the group admitted to walking a mile to her local church at the bottom of the hill every morning for 7 o'clock

Mass. As a result of the effort of climbing back up the hill she felt exhausted and had to spend the rest of the morning recovering while she coped with her pain. She felt she had to go to church every day to prove her devotion. One of the reasons she gave was that very often no one else turned up and she felt a responsibility to the priest. The group members suggested she had a word with the priest about how difficult it was for her. Next morning she spoke to him and he was quite happy to suggest that perhaps she could limit her attendance to Sundays. He would not think any the less of her.

I am not suggesting there is a simple solution to every problem. Neither woman found it easy to make the necessary changes. When they took a step back they could see how their behaviour appeared to other people and acknowledged that they had placed their burden on themselves. It is most important to question those areas of life that are causing distress and ask yourself 'Is this how I want to live?' and then have the courage to work towards change. These two women were able to assert themselves because they had the support of the group in overcoming their fear.

Self-esteem is the value you put on yourself. People who suffer from long-term illness or chronic disability are in danger of losing their self-esteem and confidence. This loss of self-esteem follows the loss of physical ability. It is made worse by knock-on effects such as losing a job and being unable to provide for the family financially or physically and becoming dependent on the state or placing the burden of financial security on a partner. Self-esteem plummets even further if the illness makes a person feel they are no longer sexually attractive and are 'past it'.

With each setback you experience as you try to rebuild your life, or when an old problem resurfaces, you are faced again with the possibility of loss and you are reminded about all the things you have lost since your illness started. Your grieving starts all over again, so does your anger and rage, and some people feel they are so worthless they might as well give up and not even try to do those things that they know can help them. Many people make a start at rebuilding their lives but because their negative feelings have not been dealt with and laid to rest, they can find themselves sabotaging their own efforts. It is no fault of theirs but it is a sign that these people need professional help to grieve and 'lay their ghosts'.

Talking about your feelings is important and will help to remove much of the confusion and negativity that can so easily dominate your mind. No one is exempt from feelings of worthlessness. They recur from time to time with everybody, whether they have a pain problem or not, but if you recognize that these powerful emotions are an obstacle to your progress then talk to your doctor about them. Your doctor can arrange for you to have psychological help through the NHS if he or she feels this is appropriate. However, seeking refuge in tranquilizers will not help to solve your problem.

Recognize when you need help

You will know from your own experience that chronic pain has a profound effect on the way we feel and behave. The whole pattern of symptoms surrounding the pain problem often gets confused with that of clinical depression. It was for this reason that every patient presenting with chronic pain at the University of Washington Hospital in Seattle was tested to determine whether the main problem to be treated was chronic pain, or depression. If the indications were that the patient was showing signs of clinical depression then that was treated first. Often, the treatment for depression had the effect of relieving the chronic pain symptoms.

Depression can often be overlooked when a person also has a chronic pain problem. Conversely, a chronic pain problem can fail to be treated appropriately because depression is picked out as the target for treatment without referral for expert diagnosis. This is why it is so important to have a thorough medical and psychological investigation. Many people consult their doctor because they feel depressed but, in spite of this, half of all people with depression may remain undiagnosed, even though depression is said to affect as many as one in five women and one in eight men at some time during their lifetime.

Here are some symptoms to watch for. If you have chronic pain then you will be familiar with most of them. They are real 'party poopers':

- frequent bouts of crying and feeling sad
- difficulty sleeping
- tiredness, exhaustion and irritability
- anxiety and feeling agitated

- lack of concentration
- headaches
- loss of patience and over-reacting
- catastrophizing, making mountains out of molehills
- low sex drive
- general loss of interest in every aspect of life
- over-dependence on medication
- feeling that everyone is against you.

You can see from this how easy it might be to give in and, on the face of it, how impossible it might seem to get to a position where confidence and self-esteem are fully restored.

In spite of all the progress I have made over the years, there are times when I step back from potential conflict because I feel that my energy would be wasted and I know that I will come out worst, the feeling of physical and emotional bruising remaining for a long time after the event. This is in complete contrast to the way I was when I was fit, when I would launch myself into any challenge confronting me. As soon as the matter was cleared up I was ready to move on to the next. Now I have to keep reminding myself daily of the things I have set my mind on achieving and to tell myself that any negative feelings will pass, that the energy will return, knowing that the coping skills I have learned, and which I am passing on to you, will see me through.

It is time now to think about recognizing and rebuilding your own self-worth and to get in touch with the real person inside. In our society, much value is placed on being able to work. If you cannot work you feel in some way diminished. In my own case, even though my chosen career was ended, I had to find ways of satisfying myself I was a useful citizen and retrained for a job I could do part-time from home. It was not until I reached retirement age that the feeling that I owed it to someone to be working became less of a pressure. Politicians reinforce these feelings when they go on at great length about the necessity to get everybody 'back to work' – even the sick. I know many people with chronic pain feel great distress and feel worthless and helpless to do anything about their situation; when they read insensitive comments about the 'long-term sick' and 'scroungers' they feel like social pariahs. These remarks only reinforce their feelings of worthlessness and make rehabilitation more difficult. However, it is not the intention of this book to attack the press or politicians. Nonetheless, I hope they will read it and understand more about the complex situation of people with chronic pain and then speak from an enlightened viewpoint.

Getting back your self-esteem

My own rehabilitation and the restoration of my self-esteem started with the pain management course I attended at Walton Hospital in Liverpool over 25 years ago. The skills I learned then are still valid today; exercise and relaxation are the foundation of those skills. Having made much progress over a period of four weeks, it did a lot for my confidence to be invited back to become a permanent mentor to other people with pain. Fortunately, I was able to draw on the experience I had in teaching and working with people in crisis.

So how do you tackle your own rehabilitation? If you are following this course closely, and diligently doing your exercises and developing your relaxation skills, you are well on the way already. When you have completed this course you will feel fitter and have a greater sense of perspective. You will value yourself more. You will have put your pain in its place; part of you but not all of you.

Even when you have finished this course try to do the following:

- Set aside at least 30 minutes each day for exercise.
- Set aside the same amount of time at least twice a day for a relaxation session.
- Practise diaphragmatic breathing at every opportunity until it is second nature.
- Simplify your life as much as possible.
- Set your own agenda. Do not try to keep up with others, especially if they are half your age.
- Know your own limitations and do not be afraid to tell people what they are. You cannot expect others to be mind readers.
- Share your worries with people close to you and work with them to sort out any problems, for example, financial, legal, medical or social. If you keep them to yourself they can easily get out of proportion.

- Stand tall.
- Find confident and positive people to be with.
- Keep visualizing times when you felt most confident.
- Do not give yourself a hard time. If you talk yourself down, then you will feel down. Say over and over again: 'I'm a great person, I'm getting better each day and my best is yet to come.'

You can be proud of what you have achieved so far; you have made a start but there is a long way to go and progress may not be easy and will take time, but the more you put in, the more you get out. As your friends and family see the change in you, they will respond differently to you and find their own ways of rewarding you and showing how much they value and appreciate you. They may have been doing this all along but because you have been weighed down by your feelings of loss, confusion and anger you have not been able see it.

Whatever you feel you are achieving as you make progress, remember that your self-esteem needs to be worked on throughout life. You may not be able to work full time as you used to or bring in a salary, and you may not hold an important position because of your illness. However, everybody reaches this stage at some time and this may be one of the reasons for decline in old age. People start to feel they need not bother to keep up appearances or host candlelight dinners. This can progress to: 'I can't be bothered to have my hair cut', 'I have enough clothes to see me through' and 'I've lost a few teeth but I don't want to spend money on dentists at my age', and so on. Thus begins the downward spiral that leads to the grumpy old man and woman syndrome. People with chronic pain should be very aware of the risks they run. It is so much easier to sit down with feet up, nibbling on chocolate biscuits while you watch daytime TV.

This is not you, though, is it? You have made the right decision to follow this course and you want to find a new direction in life, coping with your pain and not letting it rule your life.

To help you further on your way, try making a list of ten positive statements about yourself. You may find this difficult at first and you may need to think about it. You may even need prompting from those close to you. What is important is that you list those things that *you* think are positive qualities. Don't be modest but do be honest. We all have good qualities. Other people may see your good qualities but if you have lost sight of them it is time to give yourself a reminder. Make your list, pin it up somewhere you can see it and look at it frequently. Why not hang it near a mirror; then you can check yourself out, noting your posture and the care you have taken with your appearance. More importantly, you can practise smiling or giggling. Smiling does much to cultivate a positive attitude, which the American Psychological Association reports has as big an impact on your life as giving up smoking or taking regular exercise. You do not have to smile in private. Take it with you when you go out.

Activity 16
Exercise leading into relaxation

We are going to repeat Activity 7, Activity 10 and Activity 13 from Sessions 2, 3 and 4, respectively, but this time do them as one complete exercise. Begin by standing up straight, feet 23 cm (9 inches) apart and your arms hanging loosely by your sides . . . and in your own time . . . begin.

Review of progress

At the end of Session 4 it was suggested that we would be taking stock of progress so far. It will be helpful to consult your diary to get an idea of the point at which you started the course. I am assuming that you have completed all the physical exercises and practised them daily, along with the relaxation programme. You may have made a start on your food intake and the quality of food that you are eating. So just take time to write a few words about your condition when you started the course and then compare this with your condition now. Focus on your mobility, your fitness, your stamina, your general appearance, the way you relate to others, your ability to withstand frustration and your reaction to things that annoy you. What is your mood now? Are you sleeping better? Are you more optimistic? Have you begun to plan for the future? Have you made any specific changes to your life? Taking all these things together, do you see any change in your pain levels?

Session 6

The final session continues with exercise and relaxation because these are the cornerstones of being able to cope with chronic pain. Being fit and free from tension reduces pain and all the bad effects that stem from it. The first topic in this session is sleep. The second topic relates to avoiding and coping with setbacks. Finally, if you are working in a group, members will be asked to share their review of progress.

Activity 17
Physical exercise

Go through your exercise routine. It should be second nature to you now. Remember, take frequent rests, do not strain, and in your rest periods restore your breathing into the diaphragm.

Activity 18
Relaxation

Sit in a balanced position making sure you are well supported and covered by a blanket or duvet.

> Focus your attention on your breathing . . . . making it slower. . . . . deeper . . . . and if you notice any tightness in the throat or chest just swallow and direct your breathing into your diaphragm . . . . Take a few moments to establish your relaxation . . . You should have learned by now that emotions and thoughts directly influence your physical and mental health . . . Feeling angry and stressed will increase your pain, whereas feeling . . . . . . relaxed and in control will reduce your pain . . . . . . make you feel better and improve your general health . . . For the next few minutes we are going to continue with a visualization exercise . . . . an exercise that will help you . . . . . . if you are anxious, have problems with sleep . . . . . . or are experiencing pain . . . Creating images in your mind while you are in a relaxed state (this process of focusing your mind is often called meditation) . . . . . and controlling the direction of these images can . . . . . . help bring about

. . . . . . positive changes . . . If you are tired . . . . . . close your eyes . .
. . . . and imagine yourself . . . . dozing while you are having your
feet massaged . . . You can feel so much better . . . . . so much more
refreshed . . . . . . so much more comfortable . . . Just imagine that whenever you have pain . . . . . . you can enter the relaxed state and in your
mind . . . . . . go into an inner room that represents warmth, comfort
. . . . . . and while you are there you experience no pain . . . In that room
. . . . . . you can explore ways of coping with your pain . . . . . . ways of
dealing with anger . . . . . . and getting rid of any feelings of resentment
towards your situation . . . . . . or other people . . . . . . As you relax in
that room you can explore ways . . . . . . of making changes . . . . . . in
various aspects of your life . . . . changes that are helpful . . . . . that
will resolve emotional conflicts . . . . . . reduce your anxiety . . . . . . Just
take a few minutes in this comfortable place . . . . . . trust your mind . .
. . . . to help you . . . .

If you are helping someone else or working with a group then pause
for two to three minutes at this point and then resume . . . .

When you are ready . . . . . . you can become aware . . . . . . knowing
that you can return to this sanctuary at any time . . . . . . and find the
help that you need . . . . . . slowly begin to feel your hands and your
feet . . . . and when you are ready . . . . . . open your eyes . . . . . .
feeling fully alert . . . . . completely refreshed . . . .

Topic J
Sleep problems

Many people with pain complain of sleep problems. I know that at
one time my pain was so bad that sleep was virtually impossible. I
suffered cramps and if I got off to sleep the pain would soon wake
me. I was constantly exhausted. In the daytime I could not concentrate and I felt as though a black hood came down over my eyes as
I went into a fitful and unrefreshing sleep.

Chronic insomnia may be a symptom of several illnesses and it
certainly accompanies the chronic pain condition leading to stress,
anxiety, irritability and even depression. Believe it or not, a prolonged sleep disorder can also lead to weight gain and that is not
helpful for anyone with a pain problem. Lack of sleep interferes with
the hormones that control our appetite and we can be tempted to
eat too much, so it is important not to ignore the condition – seek

help from your doctor. You may be taking prescription drugs, such as those recommended for depression or thyroid conditions. These, as well as some oral contraceptives and decongestants, can have a stimulant effect that makes it difficult to fall asleep at night. Your doctor may be able to make adjustments to your medication.

Sleep is vital to physical and mental health. People with pain especially need sleep to relieve the stress of coping with a demanding illness. Sleep is a time of recovery and restoration. It is the time needed for the body to repair and replace cells. It is the time when the brain processes and reorganizes the mass of information and stimuli absorbed during the day.

There are many things you can do for yourself.

- Take a good look at your bed. Have you had the mattress for more than 10 years? Is it too hard or too soft; does it sink in the middle? Are your bedclothes too heavy? It may take some time to find the bed that is right for you. Orthopaedic beds are not necessarily the answer if you have pain. They are too hard and unyielding if you have sensitive points. Beware salespeople who come to your home to demonstrate their wares. You may not be getting the best product or the best deal and you can feel pressurized. It may be difficult to get them out of the house.
- Do not have a heavy meal after 6.00 p.m. Make lunch your main meal, with a small carbohydrate snack in the evening at least two hours before you go to bed.
- Have no more than two alcoholic drinks during the day. A nightcap, beloved of so many, is not helpful if you have sleep problems. It might help you to get off to sleep but it is likely to wear off quickly so that you wake up and fail to get into a deep sleep.
- Avoid drinks containing caffeine; instead try one the many herbal teas designed to relax or promote sleep.
- Avoid witnessing murders, rapes, marital disputes, gunfights, political arguments, sexually provocative films, hospital dramas and so on, which make up the bulk of evening television. Switch off the set at least an hour before you go to bed and spend that time perhaps having a warm bath, relaxing or meditating.
- If you have a partner then a massage with warm lavender oil is

pleasurable, soothing and sleep-inducing. Do not forget you can return the compliment. If your partner can learn how to do foot massage (there are many reflexology books on the market) you will get many benefits from it in addition to a good night's sleep. Reflexology will be discussed later.

- Do your exercises during the day but not in the evening, because it is important not to be over-stimulated before you go to bed.

- If you have pain it is important to develop a regular routine for the whole 24 hours of the day. Get up at the same time each day, follow an exercise routine, find time for relaxation at least once or twice a day, have your meals at the same time each day and make sure you get at least 15 minutes outside in the fresh air. If you can make it longer then do so, and if you can manage a walk, a cycle ride or a swim, that is even better. Try to get to bed at the same time each night. Do not force yourself to stay up because other people in the house are night owls. It is often said that old people do not need much sleep. This I dispute. Statistics seem to show that people in their 70s sleep on average about six hours a night. When you have a pain problem get as much sleep as you can. It must be a relaxed sleep so be sure to reduce the resting tension in your body before settling down. Remember, you can do this quite easily if you practise Progressive Muscle Relaxation or some other form of relaxation. Using a relaxation CD is particularly helpful. You can find out about these under Useful addresses at the back of the book.

- Should you have to get up in the night for any reason try not to have any conversations or allow any thoughts to stray into your mind. Remember, you are in control. There is no need to remain in bed tossing and turning and getting frustrated. Get up, make a warm drink, listen to some soothing music, go through your relaxation programme . . . and when you are ready go back to bed. Alternatively, remember you only want things in your mind that you put there, so consciously switch on a pleasant memory and enjoy the experience. It is worthwhile establishing a mental library of good memories and practising switching them on as often as you can. One or two people I know enjoy replaying their favourite films on their internal TV screen. Why not try? It can be fun.

- If you are in the habit of dozing when you are watching TV or reading, or if you lie out on a sofa for any length of time, make a point of avoiding this by going to bed for an hour or two each afternoon. Get undressed, pull the curtains, play some soft music and get into a warm bed. Now, just drift off. This will help you to pace yourself, restore energy and lengthen your day.
- Avoid prolonged use of sleeping tablets. They may be effective in getting you off to sleep and even keeping you asleep, but you may not feel refreshed when you wake up and over time they can become less and less effective. The kind of sleep induced by sleeping tablets inhibits the brain from carrying out its important work of psychological restoration and repair. If you do need some help getting to sleep try valerian, a herbal compound derived from a common plant of that name that has been used since the time of the ancient Greeks to aid sleep. Research shows that it significantly reduces the time taken to fall asleep and it improves its length and quality. When combined with passiflora it has a calming and relaxing effect on the muscles. St John's wort, often used to ease depression, can also be a useful aid to sleep. You will find these herbal remedies in the form of capsules or tablets, but more recently they have been developed into herbal teas and these can be bought in most large supermarkets and health food shops.

Activity 19
Exercise leading into relaxation

Please refer to Sessions 2, 3, 4 and 5, Activities 7, 10, 13 and 16 and perform this series of exercises. By now you should be getting a lot of benefit from these. As the course is now in its final session and you are about to conduct your own pain management regime, make these exercises a central part of your daily routine. It is not always possible to carry out a full programme of exercises every day but these should not be skipped. If possible, make them a prelude to one of your daily relaxation sessions.

Topic K
Setbacks are inevitable but you can profit from them

Accept setbacks

Setbacks, relapses, pain flare-ups or whatever else you may want to call them do happen from time to time. Accept these as a normal part of life and learn to see them as an opportunity to take stock, to learn and move on stronger than ever. No one goes through life smoothly. 'Some days are diamonds, some days are stone', according to a well-known American folk song. No doubt before you had pain you took disappointments in your stride and moved on. Unfortunately, chronic pain, if neglected or treated wrongly, weakens even the most resilient of us and induces a state of helplessness. This course has aimed at equipping you with the knowledge, skills and attitudes not only to cope with setbacks but to limit or prevent them. From now on, every setback will be a test of your learning, a test of your ability to make changes. Accept setbacks as a signal to examine yourself honestly and to reassess what you have learned.

Here is a cautionary tale

Over the years that he had his pain problem Fred's weight had soared. He had high blood pressure and he walked with a lumbering gait – no longer the athletic young man he once was. He had been a good patient and consumed muscle relaxants, antidepressants, strong painkillers and blood pressure tablets, yet his pain persisted. He attended a pain management course and made good progress, learning the skills of relaxation, improving his fitness with exercise and paying attention to his diet. He was an enthusiastic member of the group, always ready with a word of encouragement to his colleagues.

He left the course looking and feeling so much better and determined to carry on the good work . . . but he did not. He felt so fit he returned to jobs he had let slide – gardening, DIY, driving, babysitting his grandchildren. He forgot about his exercise, relaxation, his diet – and his limitations. The inevitable happened and within days he had a setback. He then did what many people do: went back on the pills and took to his bed. He became anxious and depressed, once more convinced that nothing was going to help him. It was a very sad Fred who had to account for himself when he returned for a check-up a month after his course had finished. His excesses were obvious to people who knew him. It was clear that he had abandoned his good eating habits and neglected exercise and relaxation.

You can learn a lot from Fred and avoid his pitfalls. Any setback is a danger point in that the person who has experienced better things can so easily lose heart and give up. In his euphoric state Fred felt 'cured' and set out to prove it to others. When a course is finished and you are feeling so much better and enjoying the benefits, remember this is just the beginning. You have to make the transition from being guided towards fitness and comfort to applying all you have learned to your everyday life.

Know your limitations

You still have a chronic pain condition and you need to acknowledge it. Get to know your limitations. Your limitations may not be generalized but may apply at certain times, doing certain jobs. In spite of everything that has happened on the course, some people, because of their condition, may still find it difficult to stand for any length of time. How long can you stand without feeling discomfort? Plan your activities to take this into account. Explain to friends you meet that you must not stand talking too long. Arrange a seat if you are going to be on the telephone for some time or standing in the kitchen preparing a meal. Accept that you may be limited in the amount of time you can sit in a car; do not undertake long journeys, but if you must, make sure you can break up the journey into manageable stages.

Here is a success story

A good example of how to manage when you finish your course is David. He decided that whatever happened he was going to do his physical exercises and relaxation daily, and he planned his day around these activities. It meant that he had to give priority to a limited number of tasks each day. In a typical day he:

- got up, showered and made breakfast;
- tidied up, did physical exercises and Progressive Muscle Relaxation;

- had a mid-morning drink;
- took a short walk to the shops and spent half an hour getting a few items to carry home;
- prepared his main midday meal and, as it was cooking, sat down and listened to his favourite music while breathing into his diaphragm and doing head and neck exercises;
- went to bed for an hour's rest after lunch;
- got up and went to visit a friend in the next street to spend an hour playing cards;
- returned home in time to greet his wife on her return from work;
- retired to the bedroom to do a relaxation session while his wife was preparing a light evening meal;
- enjoyed a quiet evening with his wife watching television.

This may not seem a very exciting way to spend the day but compared with David's previous experience he felt he was getting back to normality. He was able to get through the day without pain and every day without pain meant an increase in energy and confidence. Before his course he felt useless, felt his personality had been diminished as a result of his pain – and medication – and he was anxious that his wife might not respect his position in the home. He certainly did not want to be in a dependent state.

As time went on, David tested himself out by expanding his range of activities and doing some voluntary work at a charity shop. Getting back into the working environment for two or three hours a week did a lot for his self-respect. He still continued to punctuate his day with exercise and relaxation. He knew his limitations and he knew how to get through a day without too much discomfort. Just occasionally his pain got the better of him but only for a short time. He knew that if he continued his pain management regime the pain would pass. Sometimes he found that the pain passed if he took an hour out from activity, sat down with a cup of tea and practised diaphragmatic breathing.

Planning, preparation and pacing

Think of yourself as a rechargeable battery. You have a limited amount of energy stored inside you and certain activities will discharge that energy more quickly than others. Carrying on an activity for too long will also discharge the battery. You constantly have to make decisions about the tasks you undertake and the length of time it will take to carry them out before you need a recharge. So, think ahead, and plan, prepare and pace yourself.

Plan

Plan what you are going to do and think about the length of time you can comfortably spend on an activity before discomfort sets in. Ask yourself whether you will need help and do not be afraid to ask for it.

Prepare

Prepare yourself by getting together all the things you may need for a particular activity. For example, if you are going on a journey by air, make sure you have a wheeled suitcase available and do not pack it up to the brim. Organize the most convenient form of transport to the airport well in advance. Have items such as tickets and passports in a pocket you can easily access without having to undress. Try not to wear belts, lace-up shoes or jewellery as these will all have to be removed at airport security. The whole process of going through an airport can be very exhausting so do not be afraid to ask for wheelchair assistance when you book. If you have assistance then you usually get a seat with more legroom. This may be an extreme example but the same thought and preparation should go into any activity you choose to do, whether it is cooking a meal, supermarket shopping, simple DIY jobs or a day out in the car.

Pace yourself

Pace yourself through every activity you tackle; break every activity into manageable chunks. You must decide how long you will take over each activity – do not let anyone else decide for you; no one else should be allowed to set your timetable. Once you start, do not get carried away by enthusiasm for the task and be tempted to extend the time you set yourself. Quit while you are winning.

Planning, preparation and pacing are the keys to success for everything that you do.

Things to avoid

- sitting around watching too much TV at the expense of exercise
- lounging stretched out on a sofa
- retreating to bed as soon as you feel your pain coming on
- eating too much or eating the wrong kind of food
- doing too much for too long; whatever you do, do not get overtired
- indulging in negative thinking
- remaining in a stressful situation or allowing another person to cause you stress without doing something about it
- making yourself a martyr or a doormat
- drinking or smoking too much
- being dependent on medication.

No one can go through life without experiencing stressful events such as illness or death in the family, marriage breakdown, loss of job, moving house – the list is endless. Everybody tolerates stressful events differently. Some throw up their hands in panic at the slightest thing, others accept the situation and outwardly appear calm and unflustered. However you react to such unavoidable events, your pain is likely to be affected. In such circumstances you cannot escape from the situation; you are a part of it. It is times like this that will test you to the limits. You may be able to cope very well during a crisis, but then comes the reaction, and this is when you need to draw on your inner reserves to get you through. The skills you have learned and practise every day are strengthening your inner resources to use in any challenging situation.

Fortunately, although some of these events are unavoidable, there are many setbacks that are avoidable, and perhaps self-inflicted. It is always useful to have someone who understands your situation to talk to during dangerous setback periods. Such a person can help you discover why you have strayed off the straight and narrow, examine your situation honestly and perhaps even slap your wrist. You are looking to someone who will encourage you to return to your pain management techniques. It is not helpful to have someone around you who encourages you to wallow in your pain and adopt the role of an invalid. By taking small steps and following the principles you have learned on the course, you can get more enjoyment and satisfaction than most people. Try to look upon your pain and the skills you have learned as providing an opportunity to move on to better things.

> Setbacks generally occur less frequently, are less severe and shorter if you continue to practise pain management techniques every day.

A note to group leaders

This is the time to get some feedback from the group members. You will remember that at the end of Session 5 they were asked to make their own assessment of the progress they have made on the course. Ask each member to share with you and their colleagues what they have recorded about their experience.

CONGRATULATIONS!

You have completed this course and you have every right to be proud of yourself. Continue to make use of your skills and knowledge and make progress towards enjoying a life no longer dominated by pain.

What you do influences the way you feel. You must take responsibility to change the way you feel by adjusting your behaviour so that at all times you feel as comfortable as you possibly can.

Try to resist using your pain as an excuse not to do things.

Gradually work out ways of doing things more easily. Rather than avoiding things that you feel may cause you discomfort, take the risk – do them – *enjoy them*. If you get pain as a result – *do not complain*.

Do not allow other people to stop you leading an independent life.

Use your pain management skills every day, even when you feel very fit. Do not wait for pain or setbacks before you start to practise them.

You do not have to walk alone

Never feel that you are abandoned. From time to time you may need help from your doctor or the NHS in the form of adjustment of medication or perhaps physiotherapy and *always consult your doctor if the nature of your pain changes*. Listen to your body. You should bear in mind that resources are limited and you may have to wait some time, or get fewer appointments than you feel you need. It can be very expensive seeking help outside the NHS, especially if you entertain the hope of a complete cure. Once you have chronic pain you will always have it. This is why we must constantly boost our inner resources, keep as fit and healthy as possible and aim for the best quality of life that we can. The following information describes the kind of help available and I am sure your medical adviser will be only too pleased to discuss any of these with you. Just let me say that it is not unusual nowadays for doctors to recommend a complementary therapist to their patients. On occasions I have benefited from help from various medical and complementary practitioners, and before I retired as a psychotherapist and hypnotherapist I was able, in my turn, to help many people with pain.

Electrical stimulation

Transcutaneous electrical nerve stimulation (TENS) involves stimulating tissue with an electric current. The device used is small, about the size of a mobile phone, and is usually referred to as a TENS machine. You have no need to be frightened about the idea of electric current. The amount transmitted is mild and painless. The current is conveyed along thin wires through patches placed on the skin, to stimulate specific nerves. The current generates heat, which helps relieve muscle pain and promote circulation. It is also believed to stimulate the production of natural painkillers. The device has been widely used for many years for the relief of pain and is somewhat of an advance on the electric eels the Romans used for the same purpose. As far back as the period between the two world wars, a patented hand-cranked electrical stimulation machine, which required you to hold two brass electrodes in your hands while someone else turned the handle, was widely advertised for the relief of headaches.

TENS can be very helpful in childbirth and people with chronic pain have also benefited from its use. It is still recommended to people who attend pain clinics. However, it is not suitable for everyone and generally the pain clinic will lend a machine to a patient for about six weeks to see how they get on with it. Under the rules of the NHS the machine cannot be prescribed in the same way that drugs are prescribed and patients wishing to use a TENS machine must buy their own. This seems to me a silly rule as it could save the NHS a considerable amount of money that would otherwise be spent on drugs. Furthermore, unlike drug treatment, there are no dangerous and uncomfortable side effects, the treatment of which can be extremely costly. Until recently, TENS machines were rather expensive but now they can be bought on the Internet and some high-street chemists for under £20. I used one every day for about 17 years and was grateful for the pain relief it gave as I am allergic to all painkillers based on aspirin. Fortunately, the continuous use of pain management techniques means that I now need to use it only occasionally, when I am subjecting myself to additional demands such as going on long journeys, when I might have to sit or stand for long periods. The TENS machine is not recommended to be used when driving. Neither is it recommended for people who have pacemakers fitted.

Acupuncture

Acupuncture is an ancient Chinese system of medicine that involves inserting fine needles at specific points on the body. It is generally safe, with few adverse effects. A number of pain clinics in the UK use acupuncture as a form of treatment. In recent years it has become almost a mainstream treatment, used in many hospitals. Research has revealed that acupuncture produces benefits in a number of medical conditions, including pain. It has an effect on the brain and nerves and can stimulate the production of endorphins, the body's natural pain-relieving chemicals.

Acupressure is an alternative form of treatment, which does not involve the use of needles but instead uses finger pressure on the same points that needles are usually inserted.

Chiropractic

Chiropractic manipulation, developed about 150 years ago, focuses on musculoskeletal disorders, and research indicates that it is very effective in cases of low back pain. The idea of chiropractic treatment is that the body has a natural ability to keep itself healthy and this is helped if normal nerve function can be restored. Misaligned vertebrae interfere with nerve function, so treatment involves using the hands to move vertebrae into their proper positions. People with recurring headaches and fibromyalgia, as well as low back pain, may also be helped. I have a chiropractic check-up once or twice a year, particularly following times when I have stumbled or tripped. Stumbling is one of the consequences of spinal stenosis and the jarring can exacerbate the problems caused by narrow nerve canals, which are characteristic of the condition. The treatment effectively eases the pressure on the nerves.

Massage

A wide variety of styles and techniques exist to manipulate muscles, ligaments and other soft tissue. The aim of massage is to relieve muscle tightness and spasms, increase blood flow, stimulate or relax the nervous system and release toxic substances from the body in order to reduce stress. It is used frequently for pain relief. It can be practised by a qualified massage therapist or a physiotherapist. Massage techniques are easy to learn and research has shown that massage practised by couples on each other, or self-massage, can relieve pain.

You may benefit from using a spa. I have no experience of using them in the UK but have visited several thermal treatment centres when I have been holidaying in France. It is an accepted form of treatment in the French healthcare system, which reimburses French citizens the costs of attendance over a period of three weeks, once a year. Research indicates that this is a very effective form of treatment for those with painful conditions and arthritis. It is normal for people undertaking 'le cure' to be assessed by a doctor, who determines at the outset how many sessions they are likely to need. Sometimes it is possible for visitors to book a day or half-day taster session or select a series of treatments on an ad hoc basis without the need to see a doctor. The treatment centres are in areas where there are hot springs, the water from which is used for the purposes of massage, hydrotherapy and applications of hot mud. I found the experience most pleasant and highly effective and, 12 years later, I am still feeling the benefits.

Those taking 'le cure' can often find discounts at local hotels and guesthouses and free transport to and from the thermal centre.

Biofeedback

Biofeedback machines are used in clinical settings to help in the diagnosis and treatment of a number of medical conditions, such as chronic pain, without the use of drugs. Biofeedback involves the use of electronic instruments that measure a number of physiological functions, such as pulse rate, muscle tension and brainwave activity. It also measures the galvanic skin response, that is, how much the sweat on the surface of your skin changes its resistance to electrical impulses. When people are tense, stressed, excited or having worrying thoughts, the amount of sweat produced is altered.

Measurements are taken by sensors usually attached to the fingertips. The machine gives out either a visual display or a sound signal as changes take place. With guidance, patients pay attention to the signals and gradually learn to alter their responses, usually by altering their breathing pattern or controlling their thoughts. Versions of the biofeedback machine have been designed for home use for educational, entertainment and leisure purposes. I use one which links to my computer and takes me step by step through deep breathing exercises and guided meditations. It is a very useful aid for my own relaxation and pain control, but I also find it very entertaining because my progress is indicated as I successfully complete a series of challenges similar to video games. The only way to win is to breathe properly and relax completely. In this way I am trained to change my physiological responses, and consequently my pain, without effort.

When I was working with patients I often used a simple biofeedback machine to help those who were unsure of hypnotherapy to understand how they could be in control of their responses without the intervention of a therapist. Biofeedback is a relaxation technique that is scientifically proven to have a powerful positive effect on your emotional and physical well-being, and is also an effective form of treatment for pain. Just a note of caution: if you are using a machine for the first time without guidance it is easy to become impatient and try too hard, especially if the machine emits audio signals. When this happens, relaxation does not happen. The whole essence of the machine is that you learn to adopt a slow, deep, breathing rhythm so do not be discouraged. There is a wide range of machines available to the public and the Internet is a good place to start your search. Some machines can be quite expensive but the cost compares favourably with the cost of, say, a private visit to the dentist.

Meditation

Throughout history, meditation has been practised in Asia and the Far East and is a major part of yoga, the martial arts and Buddhism. By focusing their thoughts, people can achieve inner peace and enlightenment. There are many ways to meditate and the practice results in physical relaxation and a quietening of the mind. Scientists have noted that experienced meditators are able to control physical functions previously thought to be outside conscious awareness, such as heart rate, blood pressure and the production of hormones that combat stress or pain. Herbert Benson, Professor of Medicine at Harvard University, called the physiological changes produced during meditation 'the relaxation response'. This response is common to all practices that induce deep relaxation.

Meditation is easy to learn and requires no special equipment or clothing. It is even possible to practise meditation in situations that can normally be distracting, for example noisy or crowded places. Regular meditation practice leads to enhanced concentration, alertness and mental proficiency, as well as lowered blood pressure and heart rate and reduced pain. An eight-week study at Duke University in North Carolina, USA in 2005 showed that a form of Buddhist meditation produced significant improvements in 43 patients with low back pain. Other studies have shown that meditation by patients with chronic pain produced improvements that lasted for up to four years after training. In this book, the paragraphs relating to relaxation techniques could just as easily have been called meditation techniques.

Hypnotherapy

For the last 50 or 60 years hypnotherapy has been accepted by the medical profession as a legitimate therapeutic procedure. It is used in many hospitals and in dentistry. The practice of hypnosis has in the past been associated with stage entertainment, usually showing people making fools of themselves under what is claimed to be a hypnotic state. Therapeutic hypnosis stresses that people in the hypnotic state remain under their own control at all times. During therapy, a hypnotized person enters a state of altered consciousness, guided by the therapist. A similar state is achieved if a person is practising visualization, meditation or even daydreaming. Under the hypnotic state a person is less likely to resist suggestions for change and more likely to take on board helpful ideas for improvement.

Hypnotherapy has been found useful in treating undesirable behaviour or habits such as phobias, uncontrollable anger, smoking and food or sugar addiction, as well as in managing emotional and psychological problems. It is particularly useful in the treatment of various medical conditions such as eczema, and in the relief of chronic pain. When working with chronic pain patients I always found it worthwhile to teach them self-hypnosis. The relaxation activities in this book will have given you some experience of learning and applying the skill of self-hypnosis.

Reflexology

First practised by the ancient Egyptians and Chinese, therapeutic foot or hand massage, called reflexology, is a popular non-invasive complementary therapy. It is based on the principle that the reflexes found in areas of the hands and feet correspond to all the organs, systems and glands in the body. If you look at any book on reflexology you will see an illustration showing the feet as a miniature map of the whole body. While effective in treating a wide range of conditions, reflexology does not set out to heal specific illnesses.

The aim of reflexology treatment is to produce in the body a state of relaxation and to restore balance between the different systems of the body. The therapist uses fingers and thumbs to apply gentle pressure. Through this pressure it is possible to detect tiny deposits and imbalances. Working on these points enables the therapist to release blockages, restore the flow of energy and assist in the restoration of balance between the various body systems. As a result, tension and stress can be eased, sleep patterns improved and pain levels reduced. From my own experience and that of others, I know it can induce deep relaxation. Anyone undergoing the treatment should not make any plans for the rest of the day. I fall into a deep sleep for several hours following each treatment and wake up thoroughly refreshed and pain-free for weeks at a time. I cannot guarantee that this will happen every time and to every person. Everyone will react in their own way to the treatment and it may not be suitable for everyone, but it is worth a try.

Spiritual healing

This is not to be confused with spiritualism or the dramatic exhibitions of 'healing' that you may see on television. The patient is not asked to have any religious faith. Practitioners neither advertise nor charge for their services although they will accept donations. Spiritual healers believe that all healing comes from within and that they act merely as a 'channel' to enable a person to heal themselves. They are most effective in removing emotional blockages to healing, removing anxiety in the patient and their loved ones. This results in a surge of energy and feelings of well-being.

Healers are often said to have 'healing hands', which generate heat in the parts of the patient's body that are being treated. The hands are also used to scan the body for imbalances. The healer might detect energy blockages and leave their hands on the body for a while to promote release. In working closely with the patient the healer might become aware of emotional blockages that need to be released. There are many techniques that might be used, including powerful visualizations. A healer was part of the therapeutic team on the pain management course at Walton Hospital in Liverpool and was acknowledged by all to be a real help in the treatment of chronic pain.

Osteopathy

Osteopathy was developed in the USA in the middle of the nineteenth century. The discipline is based on the idea that the musculoskeletal system is central to the health and well-being of the body. By correcting problems in the body's structure, using manipulation, the body's ability to function and to heal itself can be greatly improved. Misalignment in the body's structure may result from muscle injuries, tension and poor posture and may also impair health by blocking the free flow of blood and lymphatic fluids. The osteopathic manipulation is designed to increase mobility and release muscle tension. Research indicates that people with low back pain and arthritis treated with osteopathy need fewer pain relievers and anti-inflammatory drugs than those people who are treated conventionally.

Having read the above descriptions you will have no doubt gathered that 'all roads lead to Rome' inasmuch as successful treatment produces deep relaxation and a calm mind – the very essence of this handbook.

This survey of complementary treatments does not cover everything on offer, but details those most commonly available throughout the country. Many people choose a therapist through word of mouth but you would be wise to consult the Institute for Complementary and Natural Medicine, whose address is at the end of the book. The Institute keeps a register of all qualified complementary practitioners. If you choose a complementary practitioner then make sure you do not agree to have treatment on an open-ended basis. At the outset make it clear that you would like to try no more than three treatment sessions. Three sessions should give a clear indication whether or not you are getting any benefit. The words: 'I would like to see you again next week/next month', should be a prompt for you to be asking how many treatments the practitioner anticipates you will need before you feel any benefit. The same applies to all medical consultants. Open-ended commitments can cost you a lot of money and may not necessarily be helpful. When arranging an appointment, be sure to enquire whether the therapist is experienced in the treatment of chronic pain.

Appendix – Using the course in a group setting

This section of the book is intended for anyone who wishes to use the pain management programme in a group setting. It offers guidance on how to tailor this course according to the number of days and time you have available each day, and advises on planning and working with the group.

There are many self-help groups that have been established over the years to provide services to people with chronic pain. Very few follow a systematic educational programme that gives an opportunity for members to work directly on their pain by learning the skills of self-management. Some may involve large or small groups of people meeting monthly to socialize, listen to an invited speaker, join in some activity or make visits to places of interest. The members may offer mutual support to each other, either face to face or by telephone or Internet.

No group can carry on its work satisfactorily unless it is fully accepted by the community in which it operates. The initial work of gaining acceptance, and therefore being able to start up, takes a great deal of time and energy. People with pain who may be full of enthusiasm but also may be short on energy would therefore do well to enlist the help of able-bodied supporters. However, this should not discourage small groups of people with pain getting together and following the programme outlined in this book. They need not follow the whole programme but perhaps just meet regularly to do the physical exercises and the relaxation sessions, just as long as the conversation is not dominated by talk of pain. *Talk of pain only serves to reinforce it.*

This way of working in a group would be helpful to people living in retirement communities or residential homes, where there is usually a communal area that could be used. People with chronic pain have specific problems and their pain should be addressed simply and directly. Learning to exercise in appropriate ways and mastering the skills of relaxation are not difficult. There is no magic in doing these things, yet they are the most important activities for people with chronic pain problems. On a practical note, the relaxation programmes can be delivered by a group member at a slow pace and observing the pauses written into the text, or they can be recorded. Alternatively, relaxation CDs can be obtained from Pain Association Scotland.

Anyone thinking about setting up a self-help group should not be daunted by the apparent complexity of the task. It is always possible to start in a small way. Arrange meetings for a couple of hours each week, focusing on gentle exercise and relaxation before tackling anything more ambitious. All too often, self-help groups start up and offer little more to their members than tea and sympathy. This service may be useful in its own way but it does nothing to address people's pain problems. People may make pleasant contacts and friendships but if the group does not satisfy the majority, the membership falls away.

Most retirement communities offer a weekly coffee morning for residents to get to know each other but very few offer structured courses. I know that some establishments offer such things as yoga or t'ai chi, as a result of management and residents cooperating, but in most places nothing is offered and many residents may be enclosed in their flats or rooms losing fitness and experiencing pain. To me, this is a great tragedy. More modern accommodation may offer swimming pools and gym facilities but I wonder how well-used these facilities are. Providers of retirement accommodation should be aware of the potential for deterioration of their residents and encourage as many physical and leisure activities as possible. Most providers claim to be helping older residents to maintain their independence, but there is no independence without fitness. In a closed community particularly, it should be possible to work towards getting a group of people together to share an activity from which everyone will benefit.

Points to consider

Numbers of participants

If you are planning to set up a group and use this programme then you will have to take note of some constraints. An ideal number of members is somewhere between eight and twelve. If there are five people or fewer they can feel exposed and overwhelmed by the experience, and there will not be sufficient interaction between group members to enable learning, growth and development to take place. If you have more than ten people it becomes more difficult to ensure the participation of each member. The programme requires the full participation of each member and sufficient time for everyone to be involved in every meeting. There is no question of rushing things and so depriving some of the opportunity to speak. The leader has to be tough enough to ensure a session is not dominated by the most voluble or needy. It is well worth setting out the rules for discussion in advance and sticking to them.

Encourage discussion and feedback

When going through the topics, the leader may wish to deliver just the highlights in order to stimulate discussion. To help this, it is worth having a whiteboard or flipchart so that contributions from each member can be written down. Remember, every contribution is important and should not be dismissed or ridiculed, no matter how inappropriate it might seem. It may have taken a lot of courage for a member to speak up in public.

Taking part in such a discussion can do a lot to improve a person's self-esteem and may be an important part of their learning. Remember, a full draft of the topic can be photocopied and handed out or group members may wish to buy their own copy of this handbook.

Take as many opportunities as possible to encourage feedback. You may only need five minutes at a time to have feedback on an exercise session or a relaxation session. If people have had a task to do between meetings be sure to allow time, perhaps at the end of the day, over a cup of tea, to see how everybody got on.

Timing

Resist the temptation to extend the number of meetings beyond the limit of the course. Everyone needs to know from the outset that the course is not open-ended. Whenever a course extends there is a tendency to drift and very little gets achieved.

I have designed the course to take place on one full day a week for a period of six weeks. You may wish to meet for two hours a week, in which case you will need to limit your objectives for each meeting. Anything less than two hours is inadequate and is not likely to be very successful. Further on, I have given more detailed timetables for meetings that last a whole day and those that take place during a two-hour session.

Venue

The venue should feel cosy and offer the opportunity for the members to sit in a circle and at the same time allow enough space for people to lie down with their arms outstretched, without touching. It should be quiet, and participants should not be disturbed or overlooked.

There should be access to a toilet and tea-making facilities, and there should be sufficient chairs. If exercise mats are not available then members should be asked to provide their own.

Helpers

You will need people to help you with various tasks. These include taking responsibility for convening the group and liaising with other individuals and organizations. Someone with access to a word processor and photocopier will also be needed to prepare the materials and information to be used by the group. These include the timetables, a questionnaire and copies of the topics and lists of physical exercises, where appropriate. This person needs to be meticulous in their preparation and there must be no question of leaving things to the last minute. A lot of this work can be reduced if every member is asked to bring their own copy of this handbook. You will also need people to:

- arrive early to ensure the building is opened and the room is available and warm, set out chairs and mats and ensure a CD player is available and in working order;
- be responsible for refreshments or providing the means for making tea or coffee and collecting the money;
- lead the physical exercise sessions;
- lead the relaxation sessions;
- deliver the prepared scripts;
- lead group discussions and activities.

It may be that there are professional people proficient in some or all of these areas but it is likely that volunteers may be needed from either within the group or outside. The fact that a person is a volunteer does not mean they are not up to the job. Volunteers have developed skills and experience over many years working or training for their own careers. Some volunteers have an innate ability to help others in a way that is denied to many highly qualified professionals, and their ability to communicate is of a different quality, which is recognized by other group members, who are more likely to take note of their message. The group will be stronger if group members themselves are encouraged to be actively involved rather than be passive recipients. Each person taking on a task on behalf of the group will find that their own personal development is enhanced. Practice will bring confidence.

It is up to the leader to make sure that group members are informed in advance of the need to bring a warm cover or blanket and ensure that any photocopies of material to be handed out are available well in advance of each meeting.

Sample timetables

Here is a sample timetable for the first meeting of a six-week course. The other five sessions could follow the same pattern.

Timetable for first meeting of a six-week course

Morning

09.45	Arrival and welcome
10.00 – 11.00	Outline of the aims of the course by the leader, followed by Activity 1*
11.00 – 11.15	Break for coffee
11.15 – 11.30	Topic A – Exercise is the key
11.30 – 12.00	Activity 2 – Physical exercise
12.00 – 12.30	Topic B – Relaxation – Breathing
12.30 – 13.30	Lunch, followed by free time

Afternoon

13.30 – 14.30	Activity 3 – Some questions about your pain
14.30 – 15.30	Activity 4 – Progressive Muscle Relaxation
15.30 – 16.00	Topic C – over a cup of tea, a discussion on how you will know when you are making progress.† Followed by target setting and general wind down.
16.00 – 16.30	Relaxation session

*Be clear about your aims. Each member will be asked to make a brief statement about what they would like to get from the course.

†Each member can be given some notes on this topic to think about at home.

This seems rather a packed day, but it works. The job of the leader is to keep things moving along. Preparation is everything. Before they leave, make sure members are given a timetable for the next meeting.

Have tea or coffee available to be taken before the start of the meeting. Always start dead on time. Starting late is a discourtesy to those who have taken the trouble to be prompt. Any latecomers should be asked not to create a disturbance and to quietly take their place without a fuss.

For two-hour meetings a sample timetable for the first meeting might be arranged as follows:

Timetable for a first two-hour meeting

09.45	Arrival and welcome drink
10.00 – 10.15	Aims of the course
10.15 – 10.30	Activity 1 – Be clear about your aims
10.30 – 10.45	Topic A – Exercise is the key
10.45 – 11.15	Activity 7 – Exercise leading into relaxation (in subsequent meetings build on this by continuing with Activities 10, 13, 16 and 19)
11.15 – 12.00	Relaxation – Breathing

You will see that the amount you can get through is limited. In future meetings, timetable Exercise leading into relaxation (Activities 7, 10, 13 etc.) followed by a relaxation and breathing session of your choice and include one of the topics each week, making sure that sleep, posture and coping with setbacks are included.

The timetables are only for guidance, neither is fixed in stone; much will depend on how the group copes with the workload. I have attempted to provide as much teaching material as I can and it is up to the leader to select whatever seems appropriate for the group. What is important is that members do not get a feeling that nothing has been planned. Better they complain of being worked too hard than not being challenged at all. The workload can always be reduced.

Useful addresses

Allergy UK
Planwell House
LEFA Business Park
Edgington Way
Sidcup
Kent DA14 5BH
Tel.: 01322 619898 (Allergy Helpline)
Website: www.allergyuk.org

Arthritis Care
18 Stephenson Way
London NW1 2HD
Tel.: 020 7380 6500
Helpline: 0808 800 4050 or email Helplines@arthritiscare.org.uk (10 a.m.
to 4 p.m., weekdays)
Website: www.arthritiscare.org.uk
Also provides community-based management courses.

BackCare
16 Elmtree Road
Teddington TW11 8ST
Tel.: 020 8977 5474 (9 a.m. to 4.30 p.m., Monday to Thursday)
Helpline: 0845 130 2704
Website: www.backcare.org.uk

British Wheel of Yoga
25 Jermyn Street
Sleaford
Lincolnshire NG34 7RU
Tel.: 01529 306851
Website: www.bwy.org.uk

Institute for Complementary and Natural Medicine
Can-Mezzanine
32–36 Loman Street
London SE1 0EH
Tel.: 020 7922 7980
Website: www.i-c-m.org.uk
Provides information on all professionally qualified and registered
complementary practitioners.

Institute for Optimum Nutrition (ION)
Avalon House
72 Lower Mortlake Road
Richmond TW9 2JY
Tel.: 020 8614 7800
Website: www.ion.ac.uk

Pain Association Scotland
Suite D
Moncrieffe Business Centre
Friarton Road
Perth PH2 8DG
Tel.: 01738 629503 (8 a.m. to 4 p.m., Monday to Friday)
Freephone: 0800 783 6059
Website: www.painassociation.com
This Association provides courses throughout Scotland in the self-management of chronic pain. It is the sole supplier and beneficiary of relaxation CDs recorded by the author.

Pain Concern
1 Civic Square
Tranent EH33 1LH
Tel.: 01875 614537 (10 a.m. to 4 p.m., Monday to Friday)
Listening Ear Helpline (for people to talk to others in pain): 0844 499 4676 (10 a.m. to 4 p.m., Monday to Friday)
Website: www.painconcern.org.uk
This group is run by people who are themselves coping with chronic pain.

Further help

I strongly suggest that, if you have access to the Internet, you visit YouTube and search for Exercises for pain, Exercises for back pain, Stretching exercises or Yoga exercises for pain. Each of these searches will find some very useful exercise demonstrations, which I have been able to perform without difficulty.

Biofeedback machines

A search on the Internet will find many websites where these are on sale. I obtained my own machine from <www.wilddivine.com>.

Further reading

Barnard, Neal, *Foods that Fight Pain: Revolutionary New Strategies for Maximum Pain Relief*. Bantam, London, 1999.

Campbell, Don, *The Mozart Effect: Tapping the Power of Music to Heal the Body*. Hodder & Stoughton, London, 2001.

Cerney J. V., *Acupuncture without Needles: Do-it-yourself Acupressure – the simple, at-home treatment for lasting relief from pain*. Prentice Hall, Paramus, NJ, 1999.

The Encyclopedia of New Medicine: Conventional and Alternative Medicine for All Ages. The Center for Integrative Medicine at Duke University. Rodale Books International, Emmaus, PA, 2006.

Holford, Patrick, *The Optimum Nutrition Bible*. Piatkus, London, 1998.

Melzack, R. and Wall, P. D., *The Puzzle of Pain*. Penguin Books, London, 1977.

Nown, Graham and Wells, Chris, *The Pain Relief Handbook: Self-help Methods for Managing Pain*. Vermilion, London, 1996.

Shone, Neville, *Coping Successfully with Pain*. Sheldon Press, London, 2002.

Shone, Neville, *The Chronic Pain Diet Book*. Sheldon Press, London, 2008.

Weil, Andrew, *Eating Well for Optimum Health: The Essential Guide to Food, Diet and Nutrition*. Time Warner Paperbacks, London, 2001.